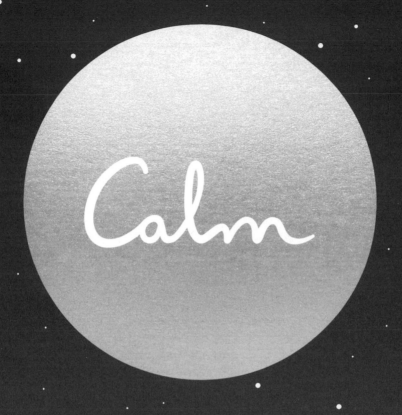

Calm

THE MAGIC
OF SLEEP

A Bedside Companion

To little Sierra, who wakes up every
morning with a smile on her face.

First published in the United Kingdom in 2019 by Penguin Random House.
Reprinted by arrangement with Penguin Random House, UK.

The Magic of Sleep.
Copyright © Calm.com Inc., 2019.

Written with the help of Nikki Sims.

Published in 2020 by
Harper Design
An Imprint of HarperCollinsPublishers
195 Broadway
New York, NY 10007
Tel: (212) 207-7000
Fax: (855) 746-6023

Distributed throughout the world by
HarperCollins Publishers
195 Broadway
New York, NY 10007

Color reproduction by Altaimage, London.

Printed in Italy by Printer Trento S.r.l.

Library of Congress Cataloging-in-Publication data has been applied for.

ISBN: 978-0-06-298948-2

First U.S. printing, 2020

THE MAGIC OF SLEEP

A Bedside Companion

Michael Acton Smith

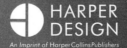

An Imprint of HarperCollins Publishers

About Calm

Calm's mission is to make the world happier and healthier.

Over 50 million people have downloaded the app and in 2017 it was named by Apple as the app of the year.

A major study of 200,000 iPhone users by the Center for Human Technology found Calm to be 'the world's happiest app' – the app that left users feeling happiest from spending time on it.

Calm creates unique audio content that strengthens mental fitness and tackles some of the biggest mental health challenges of today: stress, anxiety, insomnia and depression.

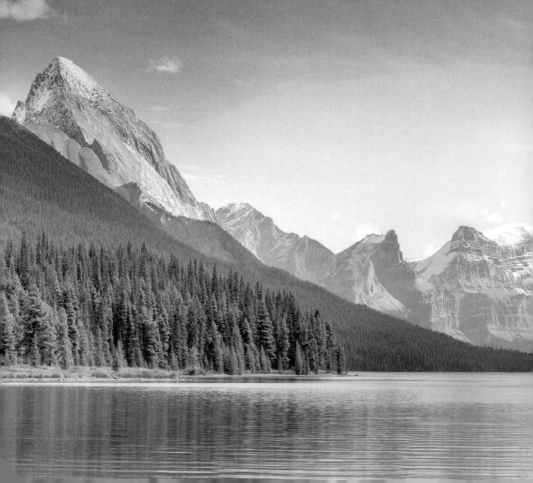

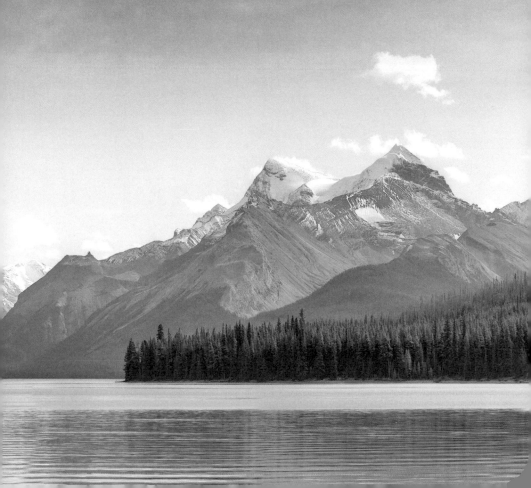

The most popular feature on Calm is a 10-minute meditation called 'The Daily Calm', which explores a different mindfulness theme and inspiring new concept each day. Calm also contains over 150 Sleep Stories (bedtime stories for grown-ups), plus sleep and relaxation music, meditation lessons, nature sounds, videos, multi-day programmes and Calm Masterclasses delivered by world leading experts.

To learn more and experience the magic of Calm for yourself, download the app or visit www.calm.com

I
love
SLEEP.
My life has
the tendency
to FALL APART
when I'm awake,
you know?

Ernest Hemingway

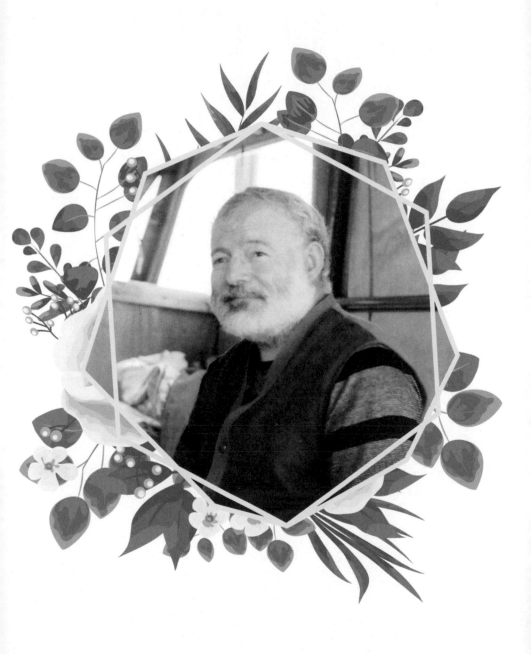

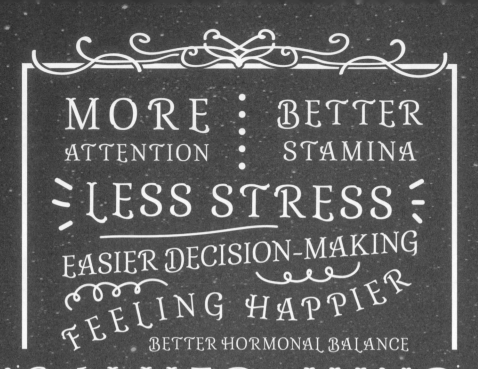

MORE ATTENTION : BETTER STAMINA

LESS STRESS

EASIER DECISION-MAKING

FEELING HAPPIER

BETTER HORMONAL BALANCE

CALMER MIND

REDUCED INFLAMMATION

MORE CREATIVE POTENTIAL

BOOSTED IMMUNITY | MORE ENERGIZED

SHARPER FOCUS

BETTER PERFORMANCE : LOWER BLOOD PRESSURE

Calm

How to use this book

This book has four sections – The Science of Sleep, Sleep Problems, The Dream World and The Magic of Sleep – but don't feel as if you must read it in this order. You can dip in and out of it, try the exercises you like the look of, or leaf through it when you're feeling exhausted but can't get to sleep. We have spent decades optimizing our waking hours, but what about the precious hours after we doze off (or try to)? This book is designed to help you develop your own, customized daily habits for a better sleeping life. It is also packed with advice, trivia, quotes, stories and the latest scientific research to help inspire, educate and entertain you on your journey to better sleep.

How journalling can help

Recent research has proven that writing has major health benefits, beyond helping you to make sense of your own thoughts.

When it comes to improving your sleep there are all sorts of mindful and deliberate practices that can help, and journalling is one of them. Whether it's tracking your sleep, capturing the content of your dreams or practising gratitude, putting pen to paper can reduce stress, lessen anxiety, boost the immune system, improve self-confidence and promote happiness. All of which promote better sleep.

Your journal will become so useful – showing you the progress you've made in terms of dream recall or in getting a better night's sleep – and as such will be a future treasure trove.

Throughout the book there are journal pages to complete and we urge you to give it a go. If you don't want to write directly in the book, copy the format to a notepad and use that instead.

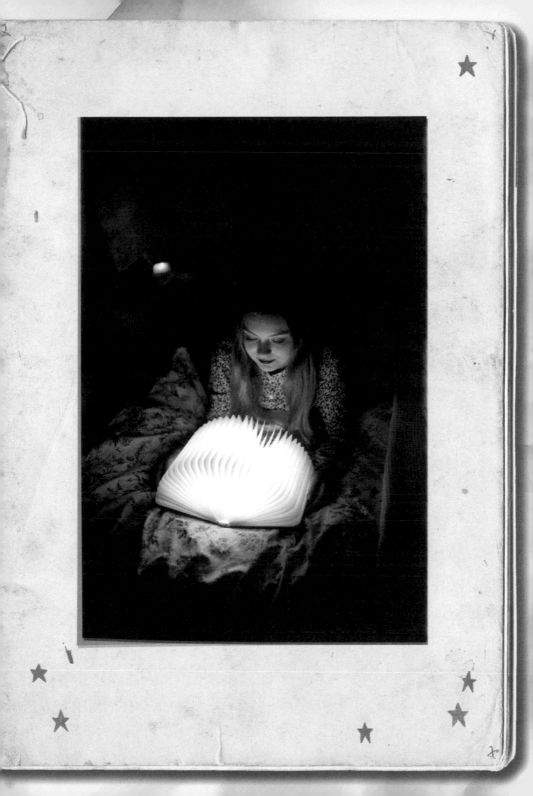

The Calm App

This book can also be used alongside the Calm app, or you can visit us at www.calm.com. People benefit most by meditating regularly, which is why our app is designed to help build this habit into your daily life. Here you will find simple guided meditations that are peaceful and inviting, with tranquil imagery and serene music. It can be difficult to start a daily meditation practice on your own, and people often find guided meditations very helpful.

Like all change, mindfulness takes time, but it won't be long before you discover that the more you pay attention to life, the more enjoyable and rewarding it becomes.

Be sure to keep us posted on your experience and progress! Send us a tweet at @calm, or find us on Facebook or Instagram where you can join the Calm community, share your experiences and ask questions. We'd love to hear from you.

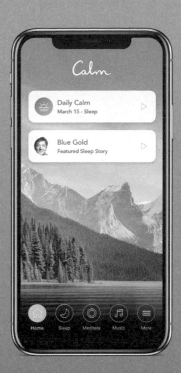

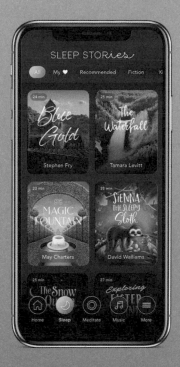

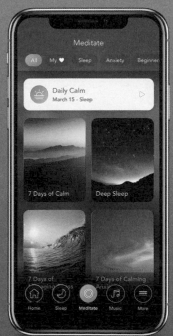

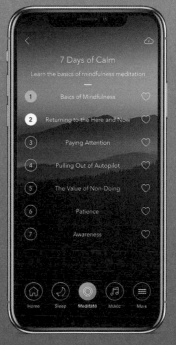

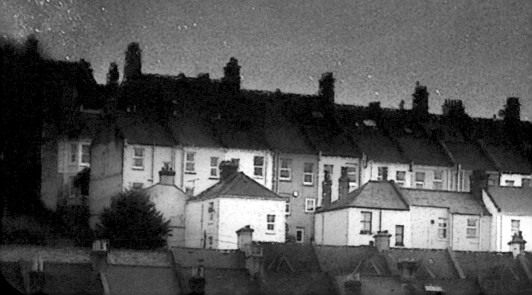

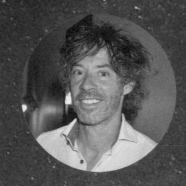

Michael Acton Smith
co-founder of Calm

Sleep is fascinating.

We all spend a third of our lives asleep, but so few of us know anything about what goes on during those eight mysterious and magical hours every night.

When Alex Tew and I started Calm, the original focus of the app was meditation, but a few years ago we noticed something surprising in the data. Every evening, around 11 p.m., there was a huge spike in usage. We investigated, and realized that millions of people were using Tamara's meditations to help them fall asleep at night. We had an idea: what if we could create unique bedtime tales for grown-ups that were deliberately designed to help you relax and drift off? We mixed in sound effects, music and the occasional celebrity narrator, and Sleep Stories was born. It was an unusual idea and a bit of a risk but the stories have been a huge success — with over 150 million listens around the world.

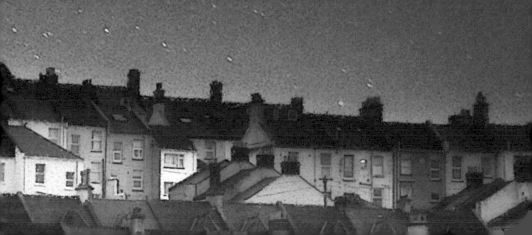

The more we investigated, the more we discovered how many people around the world were struggling to get a good night's sleep. We dived into the latest scientific research and were shocked to discover the many health issues that poor sleep contributes to, such as diabetes, heart disease, premature ageing, memory loss, weight gain, cancer, Alzheimer's and more. To shed more light on this cutting-edge research, we have included a sleep glossary towards the end of this book.

In the recent past people would show off about how little sleep they got; now it has become the key pillar of a healthy lifestyle.

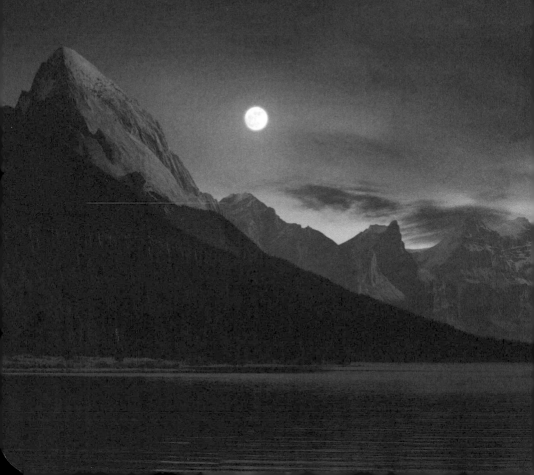

As part of our research, we also discovered many intriguing, whimsical and unusual facts about sleep that we felt needed to be shared. Did you know that sloths sleep for up to 18 hours a day, or that the two most common dreams people experience are falling and being chased?

Improving your sleep can literally change your life, and I hope this book shines some much-needed light on one of the most misunderstood but important parts of being human.

Welcome to the magical world of sleep

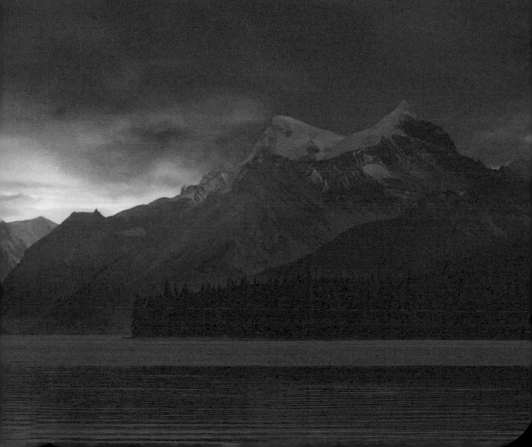

THE

Science

OF

Sleep

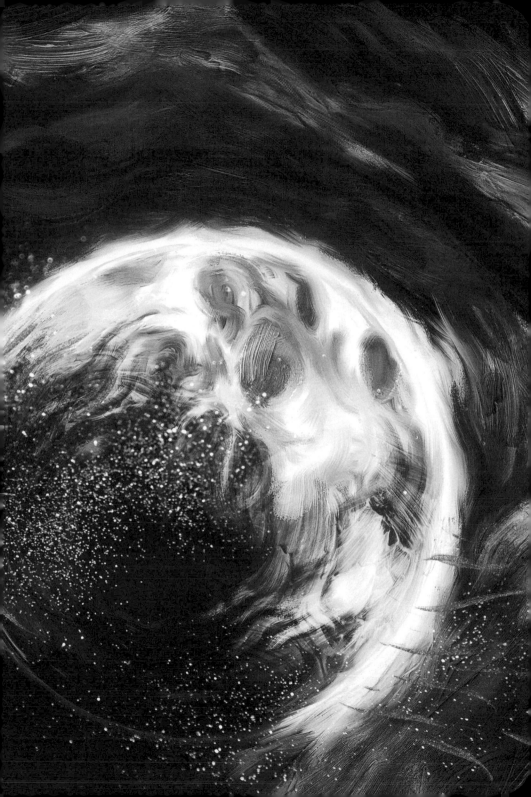

sleep in the modern world

For much of human history, we have lived by the cycles of day and night on our perpetually spinning planet. We evolved to follow a diurnal pattern – we're awake in the day and sleep at night. But all that has changed with our 24/7 societies and fast-paced world.

First with gas lights, then later with the advent of electricity and the invention of the light bulb, illumination soon flooded into every dark corner, extending working hours and hours for leisure. Thomas Edison may have had good intentions when he said: 'Everything which decreases the sum total of man's sleep, increases the sum total of man's capabilities. There is really no reason why men should go to bed at all,' but what we know now is that a lack of sleep is perilous; chronic sleep deprivation has massive implications for health – from obesity and dementia to heart disease and cancer.

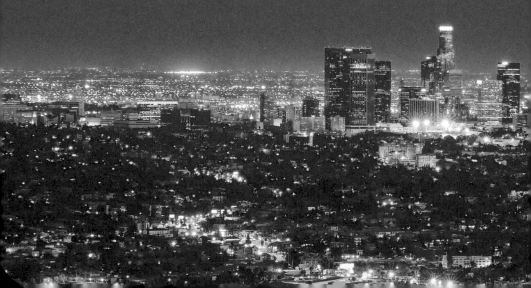

When motorways became lit by strings of streetlights, and our homes became fully illuminated after dark, we started to disengage the connection between day and night and the master clock that has long controlled our urge to sleep and be awake.

We too often ignore the signs of sleepiness because we want to finish that project at work, enjoy nights out with friends or binge-watch the latest series on Netflix. And by running on too little sleep, we turn into quivering emotional wrecks and cannot process thoughts or problems efficiently.

But small and significant changes can start to redress the balance. The natural world has plenty to teach us. Reconnecting with the sun and working in harmony with its cycle can empower us to sleep better, be energized and feel happier.

So, let's make a new mantra for the sleep revolution – let's reclaim the night for sleep.

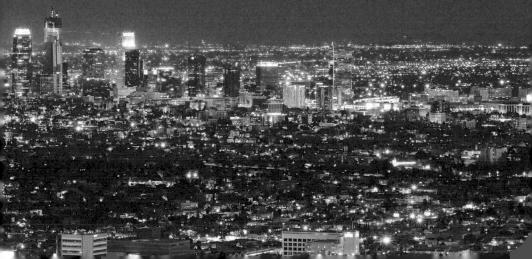

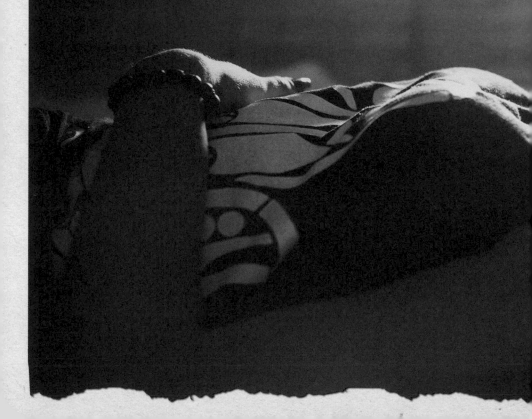

A little insomnia is not without its value in making us appreciate sleep, in throwing a ray of light upon that darkness.

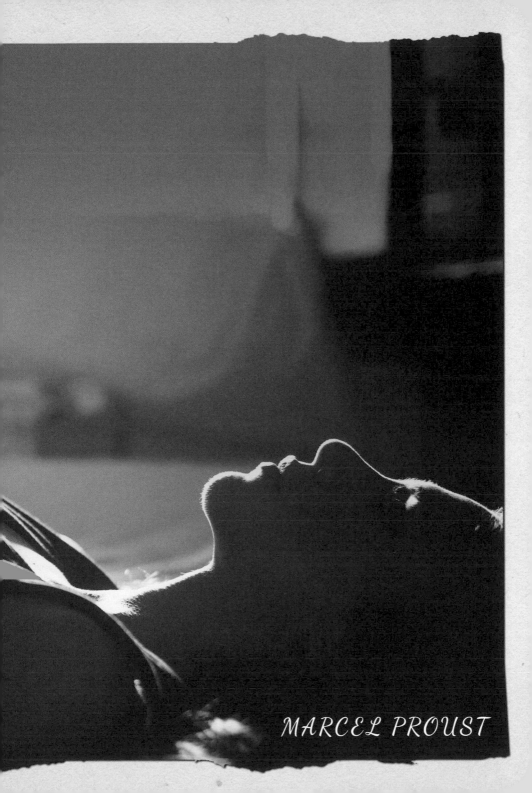
MARCEL PROUST

Give sleep a chance

It may have been an iconic protest about promoting peace not war, but we think that John Lennon and Yoko Ono had the right idea when they decided to use part of their honeymoon to stage their 'give peace a chance' event – do it in your pyjamas and from the comfort of a bed.

In 1969, the couple spent a week tucked up in room 902 at Amsterdam's Hilton Hotel, followed by another week-long bed-in (a few months later) across the pond in Canada, lounging under the covers at the Queen Elizabeth Hotel, Montreal.

Viewed by some as a blatant publicity stunt, others chose to hang out with the couple – visitors were invited between 9 a.m. and 9 p.m. – to uncover more of their peace-promoting philosophy. We like to imagine that once the press hurly-burly had gone for the day, John and Yoko settled back down for a good night's sleep.

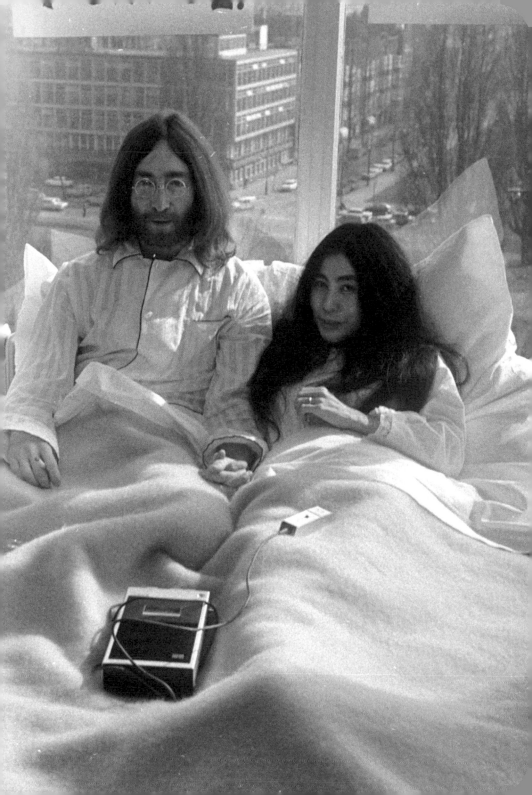

What Makes us sleep?

There are two interplaying forces for sleep – **circadian rhythm** (a roughly 24-hour inbuilt clock) and what scientists call the **sleep drive**.

Let's look first at circadian rhythm. This internal pacemaker regulates when you want to be awake and when you want to sleep. But it controls much more than that – all sorts of body-wide processes are under its spell, from mood, emotions and core body temperature to metabolism, when you eat and drink, and the release of hormones.

In an area of your brain behind your eyes sits what's known as the **suprachiasmatic nucleus** – it's your 24-hour rhythm generator. It harnesses light signals coming in from your eyes to tweak your naturally generated rhythm to match a 24-hour day. And it makes its adjustment using **melatonin**.

Melatonin is released at night: it signals to your body and brain that it's dark and time to sleep. But melatonin can't make you sleep, it simply marks the start of sleep. After peaking at about 4 a.m., melatonin levels fall off and at sunrise its production is switched off completely for the new day.

Working alongside but independently of the circadian rhythm is the sleep drive. It's due to the build-up of a chemical called **adenosine** – this compound starts building in your bloodstream from the moment you wake up, increasing all the way to bedtime. So, the longer you're awake, the greater your urge to sleep. One thing interferes with its work – and that is caffeine. Your morning flat white or post-lunch green tea floods the brain with caffeine, which blocks the sites for adenosine, thereby suppressing its effects and perking you up at the same time.

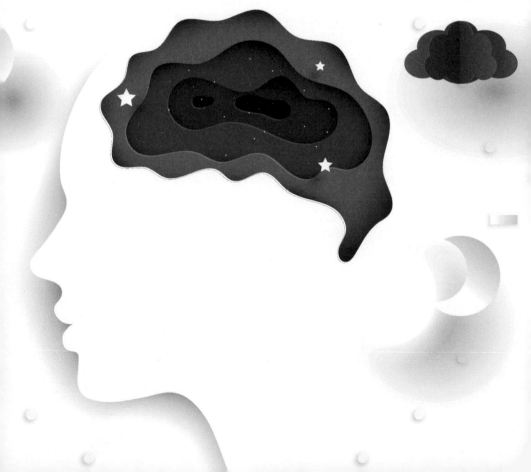

A spoonful of caffeine

Caffeine is the most used psychoactive substance worldwide, with 85 per cent of Americans consuming at least 180mg a day (two cups of coffee). In moderation coffee consumption is okay, but drinking too much, especially after midday, will interfere with sleep patterns.

How you deal with caffeine is highly personal – you'll no doubt know someone who boasts about having a late-night espresso and never has an issue falling asleep – and it's all down to genetics. Since caffeine is a common culprit in insomnia, it's good to be mindful of its effects.

Starbucks dark roast coffee	fl. oz	caffeine (mg)
Venti	20	340
Grande	16	260
Tall	12	193
Short	8	130
Cappucino	8	63–100
Espresso, single shot	1	47–64
Decaf espresso, single shot	1	8
Brewed decaf coffee	any	2–12

Monster Energy	16	160
Red Bull	8	80
Coca-Cola, Coke Zero, Diet Pepsi	20	56–57
Diet Coke	12	46
Black tea	8	25–48
Green tea	8	25–29
Decaf black tea	8	5
Decaf green tea	8	2

What's your type?

The two regulators of sleep work hand-in-hand (see the chart below) – the slowly undulating wave of the circadian rhythm alongside the steady rise and then dramatic drop of adenosine. What this means in reality is that you have a strong urge to be awake as both curves are rising, but as they diverge the urge to sleep becomes stronger and stronger; the first dip in alertness comes mid-afternoon when the circadian rhythm is on a downward direction. You are sleepiest at the peak of the adenosine line and the downward curve of the circadian rhythm. No surprise that that's around most people's bedtime.

The circadian rhythm and adenosine interplay

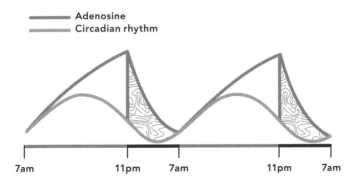

Sunlight, even on a cloudy grey day, helps to reset our circadian rhythm and tweak it to be 24 hours long.

Even 'simple' organisms such as plants display inbuilt biological rhythms.

Lark or owl? Each person's rhythm is their own.

- 40 per cent of the population are larks/morning types.

- 30 per cent are owls/evening types.

- 30 per cent are somewhere in between.

CHASING THE SUN

Today too many of us spend our days in dimly lit workplaces and we're indoors for a staggering 90 per cent of the day. Since humans evolved for foraging and hunting, much of our earlier existence was spent out and about. Despite the advent of food deliveries and supermarkets, our brains have retained a long-held connection with the outdoor world, most noticeably with the light of the sun.

To reinforce your master clock (circadian rhythm), you need to get outside in the daylight every day – and the more melanin is in your skin, the longer you need to spend in the sun to absorb vitamin D. Stimulating blue light (the same emitted by your phone) is especially high in the mornings.

Conversely, when the sun sets our brains are wired for the dark. When we're naturally seeking darkness, extra light at night is both disturbing and stimulating for the brain.

Going to bed at a similar time and waking at a similar time (what's known as a regular sleep schedule) works with your body and is one element of sleep hygiene – the term for a whole bundle of conditions that are ideal for sleep.

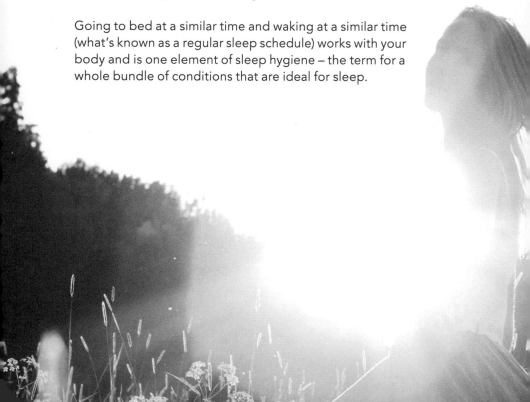

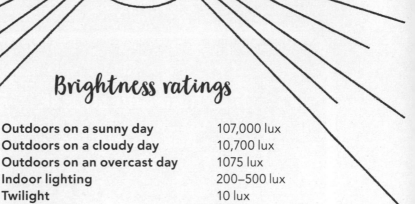

Brightness ratings

Outdoors on a sunny day	107,000 lux
Outdoors on a cloudy day	10,700 lux
Outdoors on an overcast day	1075 lux
Indoor lighting	200–500 lux
Twilight	10 lux
Candlelight	1 lux
Light of a full moon	0.1–0.3 lux

With more of us living in bigger and brighter cities, our nights have been turned to day by artificial light. So, we need to dim the lights during evenings at home and grab an eye mask for a truly dark bedroom. Enjoy a darker evening world without electricity; the warm glow of flickering candles works in harmony with your body clock and gets you to bed earlier, feeling sleepier.

Any activity that involves getting you outside in the daylight will benefit your sleep – choose a desk next to a window, arrange 'walk and talk' meetings, run in the countryside rather than on a treadmill, enjoy lunch al fresco and take a bus rather than the tube.

Embrace the natural cycle of light and darkness, enjoy the sunshine and your sleep will thank you for it.

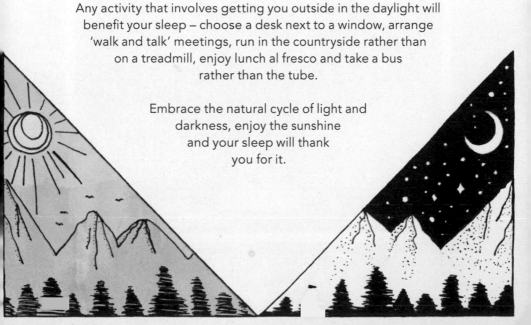

Blue light and phones, how to win

Smartphones are brilliantly useful and have become our 24/7 companions. So, when we hear they disrupt sleep, it's obvious why we've been feeling so tired lately but can't seem to nod off.

The LEDs in screens of all kinds – phones, tablets, laptops and TVs – emit a super-stimulating blue light. Your brain interprets this light as sunlight, which delays your circadian rhythm and suppresses the production of melatonin, the hormone that signals it's time to sleep. No wonder sleep won't come easy when we're signalling to our brains that really it's daytime in the evening hours.

Rather than mindlessly using your phone in all the wrong ways to perpetuate the cycle of tossing and turning, learn how it can improve your life. With the appropriate settings and/or with the right sleep or meditation apps, your phone can help – rather than hinder – your transition from the hustle and bustle of the day to the calm of the evening and bedtime.

Make your phone sleep-friendly

1 Switch on night mode – such a setting reduces the brightness of your phone's screen and filters out the blue light. If you like, you can automate this setting to turn on at a certain time every day. Certain apps, such as Twitter and f.lux, have night-time versions.

2 Set up an automatic 'do not disturb' or use airplane mode – this turns off all notifications and mutes all calls and messages. (Airplane mode lets you continue to use the alarm clock and/or certain apps.)

3 Turn off or customize notifications – some apps, such as Snapchat and Instagram, have default settings that trigger notifications to draw you back to the app. Customizing such settings can help you use your phone more mindfully.

4 Track and limit your usage – use an app like Moment, Toggl or Harvest, or even inbuilt features of your phone, to track your usage time. If you find yourself on Twitter until the early hours of the morning, it might be useful to switch off activity from a certain time or after a certain number of minutes in an app.

5 Listen to a story – Calm has a growing library of Sleep Stories in the form of sleep-inducing tales that mix soothing words, music and sounds to help listeners wind down and drift off to dreamland.

Time Travelling

Whether you're flying for work or pleasure, crossing time zones around the globe comes with a downside – jet lag. That discombobulating feeling in which things aren't as they should be: you feel tired in the day and can't sleep at night. Your watch says it's midnight but your body thinks it's morning.

Your circadian rhythm is such a strong regulator of the cycles of activity in your body that when this master clock is working against you, you feel the full force of its control. The good news is that this inbuilt clock (the suprachiasmatic nucleus) can adjust to a new time zone; the bad news is that it can only muster an hour's readjustment for each day in your new location.

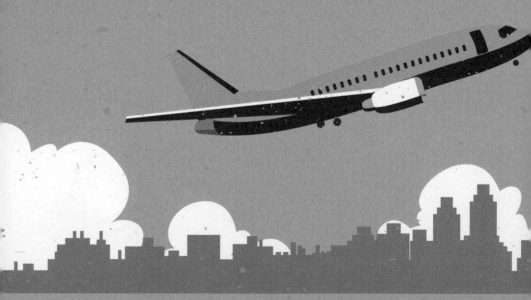

West is best,

Regular travellers know all too well that the direction of travel affects the extent of jet lag. Flying westwards, means you have to stay up later, and since most people's natural rhythms are slightly longer than 24 hours it's much easier to stretch out your day than to cut it short.

East is a beast

Heading in the opposite direction, eastwards, means you have to fall asleep much earlier than you normally would.

Top tips for avoiding jet lag

1. Be sure to be well rested in the days before the flight

2. On the flight, drink plenty of water, get up and move about and nap when you feel tired. Use an eye mask and earplugs to help screen out the light and noise on board if needed. De-stress using meditation or breathing techniques to relax you into slumber.

3. On arrival, shift to the sleep schedule of your new destination; get plenty of natural light in the day to help your master clock adjust. Try a jet lag app that creates a personalized schedule to help synchronize your circadian rhythm faster.

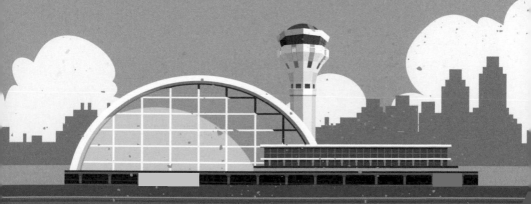

THE 10
Best ideas
INSPIRED
by sleep

Some of the greatest inventions, scientific discoveries, songs and works of art were the product of sleep or dreams. Your brain works differently during sleep, so it really is a good idea to 'sleep on it'. REM sleep, especially, is associated with creative ideas, thinking outside the box and problem solving.

01 **The theory of relativity**
Albert Einstein – **23%**

A YouGov poll of 4,453 Americans and Britons revealed that Einstein's theory of relativity comfortably topped the list of the greatest ideas while asleep.

02 **The periodic table of chemical elements**
Dmitri Mendeleev – **13%**

03 **The invention of the sewing machine**
Elias Howe – **10%**

04 **The model of the atom**
Neils Bohr – **7%**

05 'Yesterday', the Beatles song
Paul McCartney – **5%**

06 **The principles of analytical geometry**
René Descartes – **3%**

'Kubla Khan', the poem
Samuel Taylor Coleridge – **1%**

10 =

The discovery of the structure
of the benzene molecule
Friedrich August Kekulé – **1%**

10 =

*The Strange Case of Dr Jekyll
and Mr Hyde*, the novella
Robert Louis Stevenson – **1%**

10 =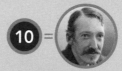

**'I Can't Get No Satisfaction',
the Rolling Stones song**
Keith Richards – **2%**

09

***Frankenstein*, the novel**
Mary Shelley – **2%**

08

**Terminator, the movie(s)
and movie character**
James Cameron – **3%**

07

The Rolling Stones lead
guitarist, Keith Richards,
kept a tape recorder by his
bedside much of the time.
He didn't even have to write
down the opening verse of
'I Can't Get No Satisfaction' as he
discovered when he woke in the
morning of May 7, 1965, that he
had committed it to a tape
recorder during the night.

'Yesterday' came to Paul McCartney in his
sleep one night in 1964. On waking, he
rushed to a nearby piano and played it in
disbelief that he'd really written it.

René Descartes, the seventeenth-century
French philosopher and mathematician who
devised the principles of analytic geometry,
famously slept up to 12 hours a day.

How long does it take the average person to fall asleep?

One American survey found that it took about 7 minutes for the average person to fall asleep (sleep latency).

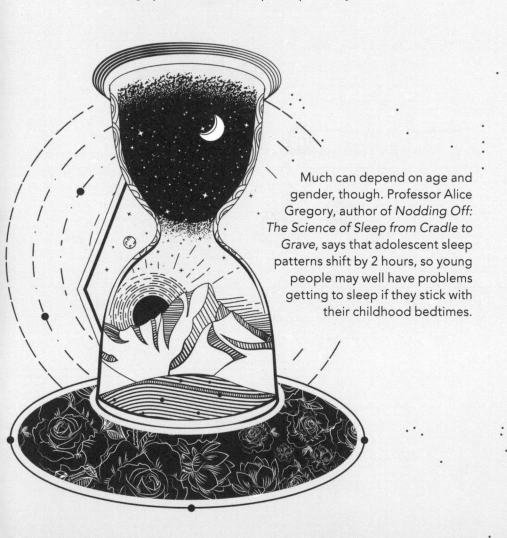

Much can depend on age and gender, though. Professor Alice Gregory, author of *Nodding Off: The Science of Sleep from Cradle to Grave*, says that adolescent sleep patterns shift by 2 hours, so young people may well have problems getting to sleep if they stick with their childhood bedtimes.

Sleep latency increases for both men and women with advancing age. There is some evidence that women have a harder time sleeping than men – though it is possible that to some extent this might be because women are better at reporting their symptoms.

Going to sleep quickly is not as easy as it might seem. So if you can nod off in the average time of 7 minutes you're doing well.

In South Africa, a study of older people found that women had a longer sleep latency than men, slept 20 minutes a day less, and were 40 per cent more prone to insomnia.

Depression and anxiety are linked to an inability to go to sleep quickly, whatever your gender.

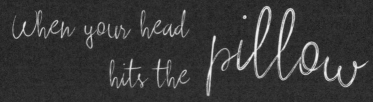

When your head hits the pillow

Each and every night you undergo a transformation – you leave your waking life behind and dive into a world of sleep and dreams for hours at a time. When morning comes, you might well remember very little of what went on during that slumber, but your brain and body will thank you for it with renewed energy, revitalized brain capacity and a refreshed immune system. You are ready to face another day.

Scientists continue to ponder what's going on during those night-time hours and what purpose sleep has – it's a huge area of modern neuroscience. But it seems every other creature also has a daily pattern of activity and rest; we're no different – sleep is universal.

Whereas sleep was once thought of as a lack of brain activity, we now know that it's a purposeful time with much going on that's quite different from daytime activities.

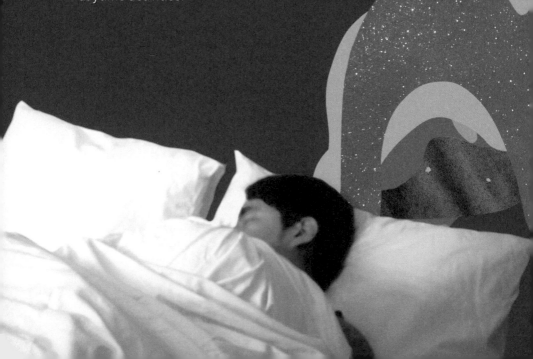

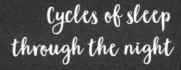

Cycles of sleep through the night

Sleep isn't a simple linear journey. Instead, it's like taking a rollercoaster ride with its peaks and troughs, not once, not twice but three to five times every night.

Sleep happens in cycles; each cycle takes you from light sleep down to deep sleep and back up again before you start the next ride. This structure of sleep – its cyclical nature – is what's known as sleep architecture. You see a city skyline when you look at the sleep graph (or hypnogram) on the following page, which shows the journey your brain takes during a typical night's sleep.

A typical night is dominated by **non-REM** (or **NREM**) sleep in the first half, with **REM sleep** (with its eponymous rapid eye movements) taking more of the limelight in the second half; scientists still don't know why there's this shift in brain activity during a night's sleep.

Turn the page to find out what exactly is going on in your brain and your body while you sleep.

The journey of a sleep cycle

As your head hits the pillow and you close your eyes, your body begins to relax and drowsiness washes over you. Within a matter of seconds after your eyes start slowly rolling in their sockets, your brain has made the transition from wakefulness (with its characteristic beta brainwaves) to NREM stage 1 (with its alpha waves). You have nodded off. This NREM 1 sleep typically lasts 1 to 7 minutes, during which time you are easily roused and may have the odd muscle twitch.

Once established in this NREM 1 sleep, you slide into NREM stage 2 with its slower theta wave brain activity and what scientists call sleep spindles; generally this stage of sleep lasts 10 to 25 minutes. Now, your breathing has slowed into a regular rhythm (and your heart rate follows suit) and your body temperature remains at a lower-than-daytime value.

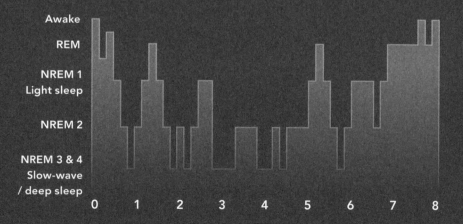

From NREM 2 you descend further into the slow-wave, deep sleep of NREM stage 3. This deepest of all sleep has characteristic delta brainwaves and lasts about 20 to 40 minutes. Your brain has shut off the outside world and consequently it's now hard to wake you.

A shift in your body's position often signals a shift in your brain activity, from the ultra-deep sleep up through the lighter stages of NREM sleep on its quest for the first REM sleep of the night. After a short transition, your brain becomes active and the vivid dreaming of REM sleep begins. Your heart rate and breathing now follow a more variable rhythm, perhaps mirroring what's going on in your dreams. Your muscles, though, have been disabled by a 'switch' deep in the brain so you don't act out dreams – such paralysis occurs moments before dreaming starts and continues for that REM sleep period.

After the last REM stage, the brain starts to wake you up – daylight signals and its inbuilt clock prompt a series of biological alarms. Overnight, the body has purged itself of the sleepiness chemical adenosine, so you wake refreshed and ready for the day.

The brain can, in fact, be more active in REM sleep than when we are awake.

Parasomnias – sleep walking, sleep talking, night terrors, etc. during NREM sleep.

7 reasons to sleep

A good night's sleep – by which we mean 7 to 9 hours – has myriad proven benefits to health. Here are our top reasons to get some shut-eye.

IMMUNITY BOOST

1. Your immune system is super-busy during the night, so prolonged lack of sleep can disrupt your ability to fend off every cold and flu bug going round.

HAPPIER OUTLOOK

3. A good night's sleep has you springing out of bed in a good mood with plenty of energy and focus. It's no surprise, then, that when people with anxiety or depression were asked about their sleeping habits, most reported sleeping for fewer than 6 hours a night.

SLIMMER WAISTLINE

2. Research shows that people sleeping fewer than 7 hours a day tend to gain more weight. Those who sleep less have lower levels of **leptin** (a chemical that conveys fullness) and higher levels of **ghrelin** (a hormone stimulating hunger). So, the more you sleep, the less you eat.

IMPROVED LIBIDO

4. Sleep boosts your sex drive and regular sex helps you fall asleep more easily. Research suggests that people who don't get enough sleep are less interested in sex.

DIABETES PREVENTION

5. A lack of deep sleep interferes with the body's control of blood sugar.

HEALTHIER HEART

6. If you don't get enough sleep, your blood pressure rises along with your heart rate. Sustain such loss of slumber and you increase your risk of heart disease and stroke.

FERTILITY BONUS

7. Fertility relies on a set of reproductive hormones, and disruptions of your master clock through bad sleeping habits or not enough sleep can result in trouble conceiving.

Quiz: are you a lark or an owl?

What's your chronotype? To put it more simply, are you an early bird or a night owl? A morning or an evening person? While it's a little more complex than this, most people fall into one of these two categories, with some sitting somewhere in between. Take this quiz to find out. Keep a tally of the scores for each answer and see what your total reveals. Scores shown in brackets.

1. What time would you ideally wake up?

   A. 5 a.m. to 6.30 a.m. (5)
   B. 6.30 a.m. to 7.45 a.m. (4)
   C. 7.45 a.m. to 9.45 a.m. (3)
   D. 9.45 a.m. to 11 a.m. (2)
   E. 11 a.m. to noon (1)

2. What time would you ideally go to bed?

   A. 8 p.m. to 9 p.m. (5)
   B. 9 p.m. to 10.15 p.m. (4)
   C. 10.15 p.m. to 12.30 a.m. (3)
   D. 12.30 a.m. to 1.45 a.m. (2)
   E. 1.45 a.m. to 3 a.m. (1)

3. If you have to be awake at a certain time, how dependent are you on being woken up by an alarm clock?

   A. Not at all (4)
   B. Slightly dependent (3)
   C. Fairly dependent (2)
   D. Very dependent (1)

4. How easy do you find getting up in the mornings?

   A. Not at all (1)
   B. Not very easy (2)
   C. Fairly easy (3)
   D. Very easy (4)

5. How alert do you feel during the first half-hour after having woken in the morning?

   A. Not at all (1)
   B. Not very alert (2)
   C. Fairly alert (3)
   D. Very alert (4)

6. How is your appetite during the first half-hour after having woken in the morning?

   A. Very poor (1)
   B. Fairly poor (2)
   C. Fairly good (3)
   D. Very good (4)

7. How tired do you feel during the first half-hour after having woken in the morning?

   A. Very tired (1)
   B. Fairly tired (2)
   C. Fairly refreshed (3)
   D. Very refreshed (4)

8. When you have no commitments the next day, what time do you go to bed compared with your usual bedtime?

   A. Seldom or never later (4)
   B. Less than one hour later (3)
   C. 1 to 2 hours later (2)
   D. More than 2 hours later (1)

9. How well would you perform 1 hour's worth of physical exercise between 7 a.m. and 8 a.m.?

   A. Would be in good form (4)
   B. Would be in reasonable form (3)
   C. Would find it difficult (2)
   D. Would find it very difficult (1)

10. When do you feel tired and in need of sleep?

   A. 8 p.m. to 9 p.m. (5)
   B. 9 p.m. to 10.15 p.m. (4)
   C. 10.15 p.m. to 12.30 a.m. (3)
   D. 12.30 a.m. to 1.45 a.m. (2)
   E. 1.45 a.m. to 3 a.m. (1)

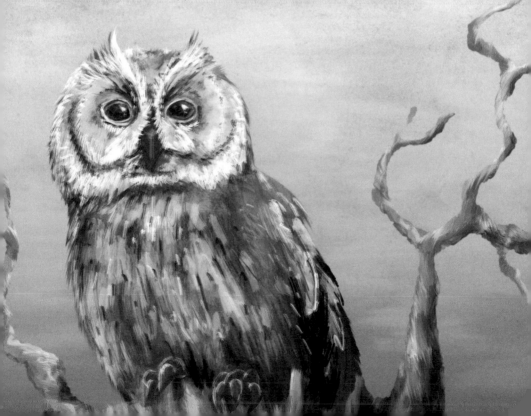

11. Which one of the four time spans would you choose to take a 2-hour test?

A. 8 a.m. to 10 a.m. (4)
B. 11 a.m. to 1 p.m. (3)
C. 3 p.m. to 5 p.m. (2)
D. 7 p.m. to 9 p.m. (1)

12. If you went to bed at 11 p.m., how tired would you be?

A. Not at all (0)
B. A little tired (2)
C. Fairly tired (3)
D. Very tired (5)

13. If you go to bed much later than usual, but don't need to get up at any particular time the next morning, which one of the following events are you most likely to experience?

A. Will wake up at usual time and will not fall asleep again (4)
B. Will wake up at usual time but will then doze (3)
C. Will wake up at usual time but will fall asleep again (2)
D. Will not wake up at usual time (1)

14. If you had to stay awake between 4 a.m. and 6 a.m. and you had no commitments the next day, which one of the following alternatives would you choose?

A. Would not go to bed until after 6 a.m. (1)
B. Would take a nap before 4 a.m. and then sleep after (2)
C. Would get a good sleep before 4 a.m. and then nap after (3)
D. Would get all sleep before 4 a.m. (4)

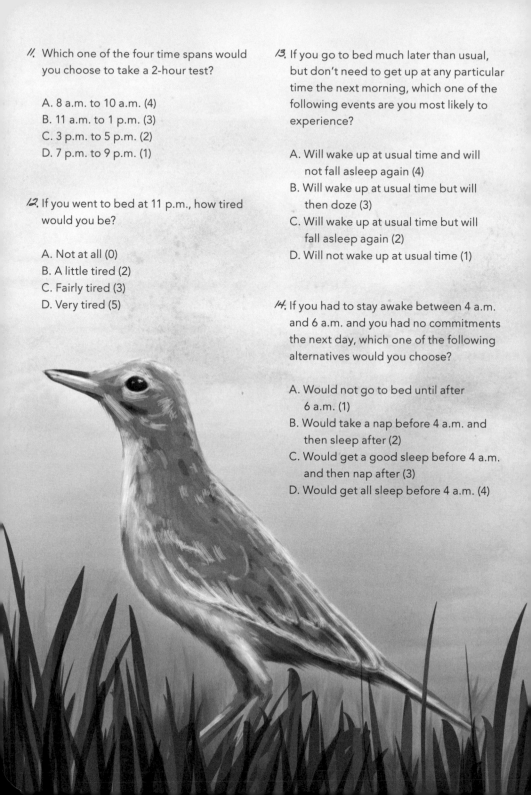

15. You have to do 2 hours of hard physical work. You are entirely free to plan your day. Which one of the following times would you choose?

A. 8 a.m. to 10 a.m. (4)
B. 11 a.m. to 1 p.m. (3)
C. 3 p.m. to 5 p.m. (2)
D. 7 p.m. to 9 p.m. (1)

16. You are planning a hard physical workout with a friend. You will do this for 1 hour twice a week. The best time for your friend is between 10 p.m. and 11 p.m. How well do you think you would perform at this time?

A. Would be in good form (1)
B. Would be in reasonable form (2)
C. Would find it difficult (3)
D. Would find it very difficult (4)

17. Suppose you could choose your own working hours. Which slot would you select?

A. From 3 a.m. to 7.30 a.m. (5)
B. From 7.30 a.m. to 12.30 p.m. (4)
C. From 9 a.m. to 2 p.m. (3)
D. From 2 p.m. to 7 p.m. (2)
E. From 5 p.m. to 3 a.m. (1)

18. At what time of the day do you think that you reach your 'feeling best' peak?

A. From 4 a.m. to 7.30 a.m. (5)
B. From 7.30 to 9.30 a.m. (4)
C. From 9.30 a.m. to 4.30 p.m. (3)
D. From 4.30 p.m. to 9.30 p.m. (2)
E. From 9.30 p.m. to 4 a.m. (1)

19. Do you think you are a 'morning' or an 'evening' type of person?

A. Definitely a 'morning' type (6)
B. Probably a 'morning' type (4)
C. Probably an 'evening' type (2)
D. Definitely an 'evening' type (1)

Score results:

70 to 86: Definitely a morning type
59 to 69: Moderately a morning type
42 to 58: Neither type
31 to 41: Moderately an evening type
16 to 30: Definitely an evening type

Source:
Center for
Environmental
Therapeutics

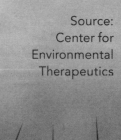

NOT WORKING 9 TO 5

For those night owls among us, even working 9 to 5 can be problematic and exhausting. But what about those working shifts, especially at night? From airline crews to hospital staff and from submariners to astronauts, shift work is a fact of life for many people.

Every system, organ and tissue of your body suffers when you don't get enough sleep. And research shows that working a night shift results in a loss of between 1 and 4 hours of sleep a day. In the short term, your memory, reasoning, emotional response and reaction times suffer, but long-term shift working is linked with the onset of Alzheimer's disease, cancer, heart disease and diabetes. So it's even more important for shift workers to get the sleep they need when it fits with their work schedule.

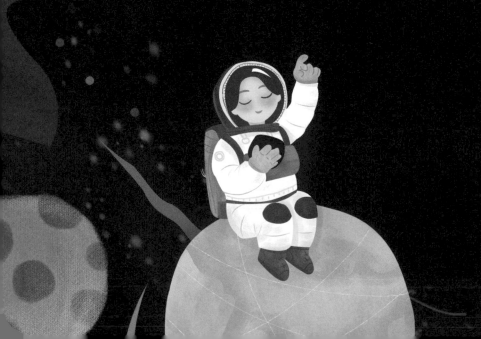

So, how do astronauts sleep in space?

Watching 15 or so sunrises and sunsets within a 24-hour period sounds glorious, but without the normal cycles of darkness and light of an Earth day, the circadian rhythms of astronauts soon go haywire. What's more, sleeping strapped down in a sleeping bag in the often noisy environment of a space station is not the serene bedroom scene many of us crave when we're heading to the land of nod. But astronauts adapt. Here's how.

- Astronauts have a strict schedule that includes sleep and awake times, diet and exercise (all of which are under circadian control).

- Each crew member has private sleeping quarters to encourage healthy, undisrupted sleep.

- Lights within the space station are super-adjustable – the colour spectrum and brightness of the lights are designed to promote alertness and circadian resetting.

- There's a 24/7 helpline for psychological support. Sleep **CBT** (cognitive behavioural therapy) and in particular CBT-I, which is especially for insomnia can help astronauts tackle any sleep problems.

- Melatonin is available to prompt sleep, if needed.

- As a last resort, certain sleep medications can be given.

First night

Despite looking forward to a trip away, how many times have you arrived in your new accommodation, be it plush hotel room, rented apartment or even a tent, and found you spent the first night tossing and turning? Subsequent nights are better sleepwise, so what is going on?

It's well known in scientific circles that birds and some mammals, such as dolphins, can display what's known as **unihemispheric slow-wave sleep**. Half their brain is in deep sleep, while the other half is awake. This snoozing style has likely evolved to enable such animals to monitor their local environment or continue to fly or swim while they rest.

Such vigilance is vital to the survival of many creatures. But people are just asleep or awake, right? Well, it appears that half of your brain might not switch off on the first night in an unfamiliar place.

effect

– half awake?

Scientists have been delving into why people find it hard to fall asleep in an unfamiliar bed by getting study participants to sleep inside an advanced neuroimaging scanner to monitor their slow-wave brain activity. The team found that this activity was weaker in the left side of the brain, suggesting it was more alert and vigilant. Such differences were evident on the first night in the scanner but not on subsequent occasions, including another session a week later. What was noticeable, though, was that when the slow-wave activity was similar in both sides of the brain, a person fell asleep faster.

It seems that while you sleep in an unfamiliar bed or place (or even without the familiar partner in your own bed), the left side of your brain behaves as a sentinel or night watchman, monitoring the environment for any signs of threats. It's not quite as dramatic as that shown in birds and dolphins, but is significant nonetheless.

This left-brain alertness might also explain why you wake every hour and just before your alarm clock when it's set to get up at 3 a.m. for that early morning flight.

Back, side or front?
The best sleeping position

Since humans climbed down from the trees to sleep lying on the ground, the quest for the comfiest night's sleep has been on. But apart from the mattress you lie on, the sleep position you adopt could be disrupting your sleep, not improving it. If you wake up with aches and pains, perhaps a new position is worth a try. The good news is you can train yourself to sleep in a better pose, reaping all the sleep benefits as you do so.

A survey by the US National Sleep Foundation showed that most Americans sleep on their sides. Yet, the number one sleeping position – as espoused by sleep specialists and chiropractors – is on your back. Next up is side sleeping, with sleeping on your stomach the worst for your body.

Back sleeper

- Good for: keeping spine and neck in a neutral position and preventing wrinkles (nothing's pressing on your face).

- Bad for: snoring.

- A pillow under the knees can offer extra support for the lower back.

Adults can shift about during sleep between 10 and 12 times an hour.

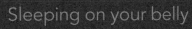

Sleeping on your belly

- Good for: easing snoring.
- Bad for: neck pain and causing wrinkles.
- A flatter pillow may help limit neck discomfort.

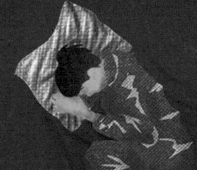

Side sleeping

- Good for: pregnant women.*
- Bad for: skin sagginess and heartburn (sleeping on the right aggravates this condition, so sleeping on the left is best).
- Choose a thick enough pillow to support your head.

Train yourself to sleep on your back:

1. Grab three extra pillows.
2. Put one pillow under your knees.
3. Arrange one pillow either side of your body.
4. Go to sleep as usual. You may find it takes a bit longer to drift off, but soon you won't need the pillows and your body will reap the slumber benefits of this back sleeping position.

* If you are pregnant or caring for a vulnerable person or child, or if you have a respiratory condition, please make sure to talk to a health practitioner before changing any habits.

THE BED

the past, the now, the future

Since we spend a third of our life asleep, the comfort of what we sleep on is of paramount importance and reflects the technological advances, and styles of a period, through history. From a lumpy mattress of hay and a bed in a cupboard to smart beds and state-of-the-art, six-figure mattresses, beds have come a long, long way since we dozed off on a pile of leaves on the floor.

3600 BCE

Ancient Persian waterbeds – goat skins filled with water offered basic night-time comfort.

3100 BCE to 300 BCE

Sloping beds of Ancient Egypt – while poor Egyptians made do with palm leaves on the floor, the wealthy enjoyed highly decorated beds, reached by steps, with a headboard and a footboard to stop them sliding out.

206 BCE to 9 AD

Hard wooden beds of Ancient China – with their elaborate carvings, the couch beds of the Western Han dynasty don't look like you'd get much sleep at all; the Chinese preferred the idea of hard beds.

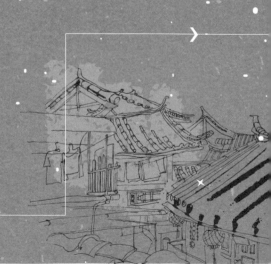

16th century

Invention of box beds – literally a bed in a cupboard, albeit a highly decorated and carved one.

17th century

The Japanese futon emerges – cloth coverings were stuffed with cotton and wool to create a plumper surface to sit on tatami mats. Designed to roll up and store away easily, these beds would be introduced to the West after World War II.

15th century

Beds with curtain ceilings – not quite the four-poster we know today, these beds had curtains just on the 'roof' and bedhead, but mattresses were likely stuffed with more luxurious feathers. King Louis XIV famously had 413 beds, most of which would have been decorated with gold, silver and pearls.

500 AD to 1500 AD

Rope-strung wooden beds – while the poor in the Middle Ages had to catch some shut-eye on piles of hay with animal skins, the wealthier class had a wooden bed frame with ropes strung across to support a soft but lumpy mattress. Sometimes curtains were hung around for warmth and privacy.

785 BCE to 476 AD

Softer mattresses of Ancient Rome – mattresses were stuffed with reeds, wool or hay, or with feathers for wealthier inhabitants.

1865

First coil spring – German inventor Heinrich Westphal patented his coil spring for beds. Sadly he never benefited from the success of his invention and died in poverty.

1895

Harrods sold the first modern water bed.

1900

James Marshall invented the inner-spring mattress – the coil springs still take his name (Marshall coils) and these little wiry bits of metal meant that a mattress was no longer lumpy.

1940s

First airbeds – with the invention of vulcanized rubber fabrics, mattresses became lightweight and more portable.

1929

First latex mattress – this mattress by Dunlopillo, super expensive in its day, was initially exclusively sold to the British Royal Family.

Today companies like Casper are valued at over $1 billion and leading the charge with their 'bed-in-a-box' packages.

2000

The no-flip mattress – no more weekly or monthly turnings needed for this high-tech layered mattress.

1960s

Modern waterbed arrives – hailing from San Francisco originally, the fad for a fluid sleeping surface declined by the 1990s.

1990s

Space-age foam mattresses gain traction – following the invention of memory foam in the 1970s by NASA.

1974

Electric adjustable beds at home – after their success in hospital use, Craftmatic brought these highly adjustable beds to the bedroom.

How did you sleep last night?

Below are some practices that can improve your quality of sleep. How many are part of your bedtime routine? Which are you not doing currently but feel are doable and desirable to include from now on?

Tick what's right for you:

Current practice   New habit to try

- ☐ ☐ Listening to a podcast or a Calm Sleep Story
- ☐ ☐ Listening to relaxing music
- ☐ ☐ Dimming the lights
- ☐ ☐ Drinking lots of water during the day only
- ☐ ☐ Regular exercise but not late in the evening
- ☐ ☐ Avoiding screens and blue light before bed
- ☐ ☐ Getting outside for air daily
- ☐ ☐ Using a sleep mask or earplugs
- ☐ ☐ Drinking decaf tea before bed, rather than caffeinated
- ☐ ☐ A clutter-free bedroom
- ☐ ☐ Keeping a notebook by your bed to record your thoughts
- ☐ ☐ Meditation (e.g. Calm's deep sleep meditation)
- ☐ ☐ Breathing or movement exercise
- ☐ ☐ Aromatherapy
- ☐ ☐ Cooler temperatures in the bedroom
- ☐ ☐ A set bedtime

Anything else?

- Is there anything else that helps you get a good night's sleep, or any other practices you would like to try?

- What else could be affecting your ability to get a good night's sleep? It may be circumstantial (a partner's snoring) or more personal (an emotional situation that is causing distress). Write these things down and explore connections to your sleep health.

How would you rate the quality of your sleep?

0   1   2   3   4   5   6   7   8   9   10

I am exhausted
most of the time.

I feel well rested and
energized most of the time.

Circle how you most often feel when you wake up.

Refreshed	Tired	Energized	Calm
Recharged	Happy	Peaceful	Enthusiastic
Drained	Sad	Irritable	Resentful
Anxious	Lethargic	Frustrated	Content

It would be good to revisit how you score on these last two sections after you've been trying to follow good sleep hygiene and have identified what works for you. Seeing results will encourage you to stick with it.

Gatherings of friends, late-night drinking, gym sessions, family lunches . . . but there's plenty of time to sleep it off, right? So, how come even after snoozes galore, you still feel groggy come Sunday night? The answer is social jet lag.

When your obligations don't line up neatly with your body's need to sleep, you'll have brain fog and feel tired all the time; it's like you're switching between two time zones (one is your body clock and one is dictated by work and social events).

Surely, weekend lie-ins can't be all bad, can they? In a word, yes. Messing with your internal clock (and everything that's linked with that) doesn't come with any positives in terms of health.

Social Jet lag

This perpetual pattern of not getting
enough sleep and being out of sync
with your body's natural rhythm has
proven links to heart disease, obesity and
diabetes, let alone the effects on coordination,
memory and emotional responses.

And you don't have to be partying until dawn to suffer its ill-effects.
Research suggests that two-thirds of us experience an hour or so of
social jet lag each week, with one-third fielding 2 hours or more.

The solution to reclaiming those lost hours of sleep? Go to bed earlier
rather than sleep in; failing that, take an afternoon nap. Plus, help to
tweak your circadian rhythm with plenty of light stimulation in the day
and very little at night.

Owls more affected by social jet lag

Whether you're a morning or evening person also feeds into social
jet lag. In modern life, owls generally come off worst, since they're
forced to get up before they're ready for a 9 a.m. start at work but
don't feel sleepy come 11 p.m. when larks are mostly tucked up in
bed and snoozing. Perhaps if employers looked at more flexible
working hours (11 until 7 could be the new 9 to 5), owls could even
up the odds and get their fair share of sleep.

Sleep habits from

Travel the globe and you'll see that sleep habits vary immensely. Here are just a few sleep stories from around the planet.

In Bali, when people experience an intense fear, they can put themselves into a meditative sleep known as *todoet poeles*. Sleep is an effective way of removing stress.

Hammocks help sleepers avoid insects and snakes. They are so important to the people of the Yucatán in Mexico that every home has hammock hooks on the walls.

In Japan, falling asleep at work is often seen as a positive sign. It's called *inemuri*, which means 'present while sleeping'.

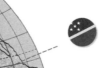

In traditional Pacific island societies such as the Solomon Islands, villagers do not have beds, but will unroll a grass mat on the floor and sleep on that.

In Australia, the Aboriginal Warlpiri people sleep together in a *yunta*, or row, with the youngest, oldest and sickest in the middle and the fittest on the outside.

around the world

In Norway, it's common to see babies sleeping outside in their prams – even in freezing temperatures. Norwegians believe that sleeping outside improves the immune system. At kindergarten, they sometimes have outside beds, including one for the teacher.

Swedes and Danes swear by buffing – placing a baby on its tummy and tapping its bottom rhythmically until he or she goes to sleep.

The British are partial to a cup of tea or a warm, milky drink before they go to sleep.

Swiss babies are put in *hängematten* or hammocks after birth to mimic the movement of the womb.

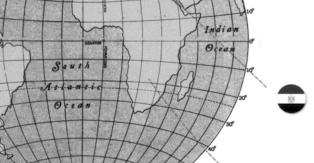

Today's Egyptians have similar polyphasic sleep routines to their ancient ancestors. They co-sleep at night for 6 hours but have an Egyptian version of a siesta – a *ta'assila* – for around 2 hours in the afternoon.

Guatemalan children sleep with a worry doll, called a *muñeca quitapena*, under their pillow. Children tell the doll their worries and in the morning the doll has taken them away.

In Botswana, the Juǀ'hoansi people of the Kalahari Desert have no bedtime and simply sleep when they are tired.

DRIVING TIRED?
take a break

The perils of a lack of sleep are many, but none is quite so terrifying or deadly as falling asleep at the wheel of a vehicle, even for just a moment.

Such failures of concentration can result either in falling asleep completely while driving or in 'microsleeps' – tiny bursts of sleep (2–30 seconds), often experienced without a person noticing. Ever felt your head nod while travelling? You may have actually had a microsleep. These momentary lapses of concentration cause most driving accidents.

During a microsleep, there is no reaction from the brain – it's not responding to any stimuli from the outside world – so, in fact, microsleeping is much more dangerous than driving under the influence of alcohol, where the brain sees the world but reacts more slowly.

Brake, the UK road safety charity, says that 1 in 6 crashes resulting in death or injury on the roads is fatigue-related. And in the US, research shows that an estimated 1 in 25 adult drivers reports having fallen asleep while driving in the previous 30 days.

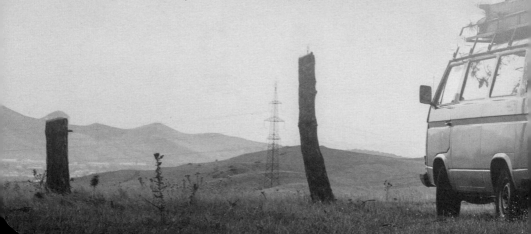

A lapse of concentration of just a few seconds, even at 30 m.p.h., can spell danger for any road-user. But it's motorways and high-speed roads, and the monotony of such cruising, that are responsible for many fatigue-related driving accidents. Such incidents peak when the body is naturally sleepiest: 2 a.m. to 6 a.m. and 2 p.m. to 4 p.m.

What's more, if you're already sleep-deprived, you're ill-equipped to judge how tired you actually are. Who would have thought, for example, that surviving on 6 hours of sleep a night for a stretch of 10 days (after trying to finish that box set) would result in the same impairment to concentration as going without sleep for 24 hours straight?

The best advice is, if you're even vaguely tired, don't drive. And if you feel drowsy while driving, pull over whenever you can and stop for the night.

Drivers are 20 times more likely to fall asleep at the wheel at 6 a.m. than at 10 a.m.

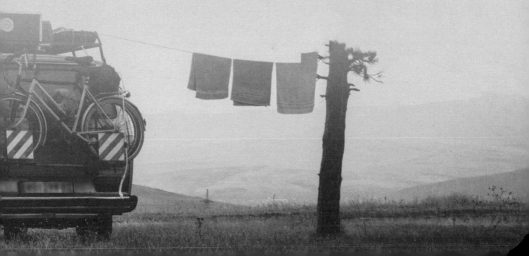

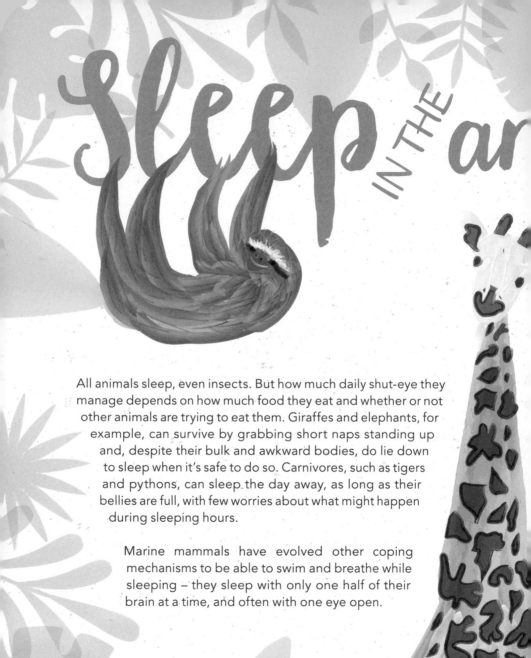

sleep IN THE ar

All animals sleep, even insects. But how much daily shut-eye they manage depends on how much food they eat and whether or not other animals are trying to eat them. Giraffes and elephants, for example, can survive by grabbing short naps standing up and, despite their bulk and awkward bodies, do lie down to sleep when it's safe to do so. Carnivores, such as tigers and pythons, can sleep the day away, as long as their bellies are full, with few worries about what might happen during sleeping hours.

Marine mammals have evolved other coping mechanisms to be able to swim and breathe while sleeping – they sleep with only one half of their brain at a time, and often with one eye open.

mal world

Hours sleep	Animal
1.9	Giraffe
2	African elephant
5.3	Goat
7	Guppy
9.7	Chimpanzee
10.4	Bottle-nosed dolphin
10.6	Dog
12.1	Mouse
14.4	Python
15.8	Tiger
18	Sloth
19.9	Brown bat

SLOTHS ARE THE WORLD'S GREATEST SLEEP AND RELAXATION AMBASSADORS

SPERM WHALES

Sperm whales nap vertically with their tails down.

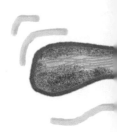

HORSES

Horses lock their legs so they can nap or sleep standing up – no muscle effort is needed to keep them upright.

DOLPHINS

Newborn dolphins and their mothers go without sleep for the first month of life.

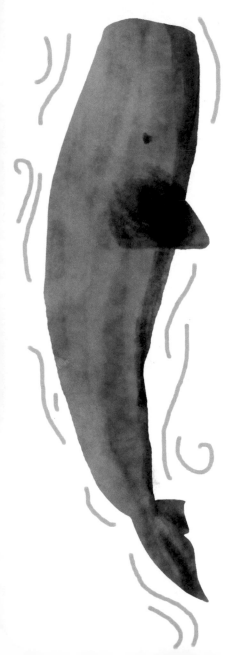

SEALS

When out at sea, seals sleep with half their brain so they can remain vigilant.

ELEPHANTS

Wild elephants can go without sleep for stretches of time – to evade predators or poachers – often for 48 hours at a time, with little obvious sign of this sleep deprivation.

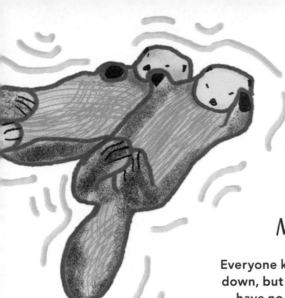

OTTERS

During naps, sea otters hold hands to make sure they don't float away from one another.

MANATEES

Everyone knows that bats sleep upside down, but manatees? These 'sea cows' have no known predators and like nothing better than zonking out on the sea floor, upside down. They do have to surface every few minutes for air, but this requires minimal effort.

PARROTFISH

Parrotfish secrete a jelly-like cocoon that surrounds them and protects them from parasites while they sleep.

COMMON SWIFT

Common swifts sleep on the wing because they spend an incredible 10 months of the year in the air, without landing.

MEERKATS

Meerkats cuddle up together during sleep to keep warm and form a protective pack.

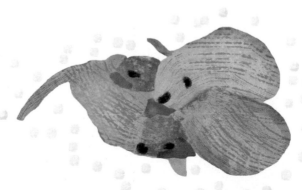

sleep hacks – alternative sleep cycles

If like Margaret Thatcher – who benefited from a rare sleep gene – you think that 'sleep is for wimps' or feel that there aren't enough hours in the day, then discover how some people break up their sleep for maximum productivity.

There are basically three sleep patterns:

Monophasic

Biphasic

1. Monophasic – sleeping for 7 to 9 hours and being awake for 15 to 17 hours a day.

2. Biphasic – sleeping for 6 hours or so at night and for 30 to 90 minutes in the afternoon.

● Awake

○ Asleep

Everyman

Dymaxion

Uberman

3. Polyphasic – sleeping several times a day in various patterns, including 'everyman', 'uberman' and 'dymaxion'.

No two people have exactly the same sleep requirements – it's about finding what works best for you. That may well be one long sleep at night, a shorter night-time snooze with a few daytime naps thrown into the mix, or something altogether different.

Buckminster Fuller – an American architect and inventor – reputedly slept for only 2 hours a day. He coined the term 'dymaxion' for his sleep schedule of four 30-minute sleeps spread equally across the day.

Leonardo da Vinci was said to follow the 'uberman' sleep schedule.

Should we all siesta?

The most common biphasic pattern is the siesta – so ingrained in the culture of Spain that some shops and offices still shut from 2 p.m. to 5 p.m. Napping for 90 minutes in the afternoon allows you to complete one cycle of sleep, so you wake up feeling refreshed. Shorter siestas of 20 to 30 minutes are also great pick-me-ups.

Before you try any of this out, know that scientists believe that there is little evidence of **polyphasic sleep** (sleep over several occasions within 24 hours) being advisable in the long run.

How to get a child to sleep – weirdest tricks revealed

Sleep can be especially precarious for parents of young children. So it's no real surprise that parents will go to great lengths to get their children off safely to sleep – from running the vacuum cleaner and watching a crossword puzzle tournament to getting the child to listen to a recording of people yawning. But the weirdest method of all? Explaining to a child the road-building plans of China's leader, Xi Jinping – the chosen method of 46 per cent of respondents in our survey of British and American parents.

1. Explaining the infrastructure dream of China's leader, Xi Jinping, to the child – 46%

2. Having the child listen to a recording of a chapter from an eighteenth-century Scottish economics book, read by a really boring teacher – 36%

3. Having the child watch a video of a crossword puzzle tournament – 35%

4. Getting the child to listen to an hour-long recording of people yawning – 34%

5. Running a vacuum cleaner in the same room as the child, for the soothing sound – 28%

=6. Having the child watch Baa Baa Land, an 8-hour slow-motion film about sheep grazing – 27%

=6. Inventing an imaginary figure, like 'the 8 O'clock Man', who tries to catch children awake after 8 p.m. – 27%

These are the findings of an international survey, conducted by pollsters YouGov, on behalf of Calm and Moshi Twilight Sleep Stories.

If you have a young family, what trick from the list will you be trying next?

=**8.** Laying the child on the parent's chest, and the parent slowly spinning in a circle – 21%

=**8.** Going for a drive, having the child listen to music/stories – and then all sleeping in the car* – 21%

10. Turning/pointing the child's bed the other way round – 17%

11. Putting a ticking clock under the child's pillow, to mimic the mother's heartbeat – 16%

12. Putting an item of clothing that smells of the mother in the child's bed** – 10%

? Don't know / None of these – 11%

* Children and vulnerable people should never be left alone in the car.

** Please always seek a medical practitioner's advice before administering any essential oils.

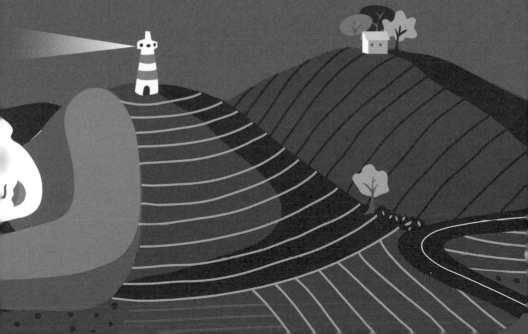

SLEEP across the AGES

From the cradle to the grave, we all need sleep. But how much sleep we require varies by age, as does the pattern in which we catch those ZZZs.

After a tough week at work, you may feel you want to 'sleep like a baby'. Focusing on snoozing is a great idea, but do you really want to take short snippets of sleep throughout the day *and* the night, waking every 3 to 4 hours?

While a baby is establishing his or her circadian rhythms, this sort of pattern across 24 hours is typical. As infants grow they're able to sleep longer in one go and catch the rest of their snooze time as naps during the day.

As their brains are developing, so their sleep make-up is changing. A 6-month-old baby, for instance, spends roughly equal time in NREM and REM sleep. By the time of their fifth birthday, this ratio has altered in favour of NREM (70 NREM:30 REM), and when the teen years arrive the balance tweaks yet again, to the 80:20 NREM:REM split that remains into midlife.

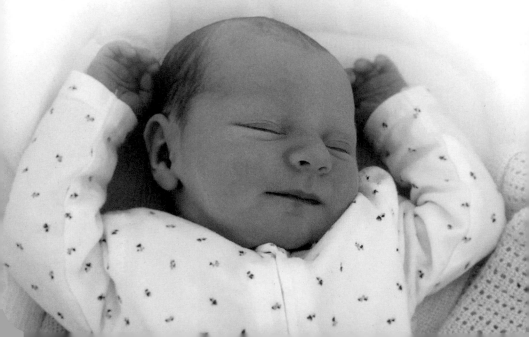

Contrary to popular belief, older adults still need 7 to 8 hours of sleep a night; the requirement for sleep doesn't diminish with age. What does change, though, is that sleep quality is affected – people have to contend with more broken sleep (waking up – most commonly for a pee – and then not getting back to sleep easily afterwards). Among the worst affected are new parents, who face 6 years of sleepless nights.

Teens – a special case

The timing of the body's master clock shifts during puberty. A teenager's natural inclination is to be late to bed and late to rise. Teens do need more sleep than adults, but their delayed body clock makes it tough to get up early for school. In the US, a few states have pushed back the start of high school – academic performance and attendance both benefited, as did the teens, with better sleep.

Newborns (0 to 3 months)	Between 14 to 17 hours	
Infants (4 to 11 months)	12 to 15	
Toddlers (1 to 2 years)	11 to 14	
Preschoolers (3 to 5)	10 to 13	
School-age children (6 to 13)	9 to 11	
Teenagers (14 to 17)	8 to 10	
Younger adults (18 to 25)	7 to 9	
Adults (26 to 64)	7 to 9	
Older adults (65+)	7 to 8	

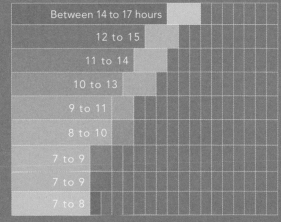

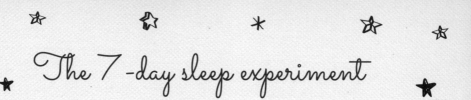

The 7-day sleep experiment

Plan to have one week clear of social events and work deadlines. For this week, the plan is to go to bed at least 9 hours before you need (or want) to wake up and to keep note of when you wake up naturally. Set an alarm just in case, but give yourself the full 9 hours.

Such an approach will help you to determine how much sleep is right for you. While 7 to 9 hours may be ideal, this amount might not feel achievable for everyone. But if you're getting fewer than 7 hours of sleep, you should work towards getting more. Challenge yourself to add an extra hour.

Plan your bedtime and alarm wake-up time for the week

The fast pace of modern life means unwinding can feel difficult, even a bit strange. But as our bodies and minds become accustomed to it, we can remember how natural it is to be in a state of calm, and how pleasing it can be simply to drift off to sleep with little effort.

Reconnecting with our bodies' biological rhythms takes practice. Getting outside every day helps to reset your master clock, but any intuitive feelings come with regularity and developing a routine. A routine eliminates the stress of having to make decisions. It settles the nervous system. And, when repeated, it becomes a new way of being. A regular routine is especially vital when it comes to your sleep.

Do you have a sense of how many hours would be ideal for you to sleep at this time in your life? Write down any insights that you have from this experiment.

How much sleep do we really need?

	Bedtime	Wake-up Time
Su	__:__	__:__
M	__:__	__:__
T	__:__	__:__
W	__:__	__:__
Th	__:__	__:__
F	__:__	__:__
Sa	__:__	__:__

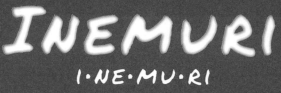

INEMURI
I·NE·MU·RI

In Japan, napping at work, in lectures, in shops, at cafés, on trains and even on public stairs isn't frowned upon – it's entirely culturally acceptable. *Inemuri* translates into English as 'sleeping while present' or 'sleeping on duty' and is considered by the Japanese as a sign of diligence – working so hard you're exhausted.

People of all ages partake in *inemuri*, a practice that's over 1,000 years old. Maybe the fact that such public napping is commonplace is because it can be understood by the results of a 2015 Japanese government study, according to which, almost 40 per cent of adults sleep fewer than 6 hours a night.

Unlike some countries, working overtime in Japan is simply part of work culture; it's not surprising to find a worker's day reaching 10 hours or more. Long hours and giving your all are an expression of your diligence, a quality highly valued in Japan. So what if you slept briefly during that meeting? You were present and that's what matters. But it's worth mentioning another word: *karōshi*. In Japanese, this describes death from overwork, which could be a consequence of continuous sleeplessness.

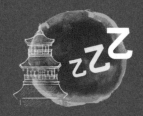

'I have left orders to be awakened at any time in case of national emergency, even if I'm in a cabinet meeting.'

– Ronald Reagan

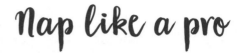

nap like a pro

Hit that afternoon slump? Then take a nap. This short sleep can re-energize you, help to strengthen your memory and even cut your risk of heart disease. So, channel your inner cat to snatch a daytime snooze.

The urge to nap is strongest after lunch, due to the combination of your circadian rhythms and your sleep drive. So an ideal nap time for many is between 2 p.m. and 3 p.m. But leave it later than 4 p.m. and your night-time sleep will suffer.

Short sleeps include light sleep only – enjoy a nap for 30 minutes or more and you slip into the realm of deeper slumber. It's harder waking from this sleep and you'll feel groggy – what's known as sleep inertia – for up to half an hour afterwards.

Cats may look like they're sleeping all the time – some can sleep up to 20 hours a day – but, in fact, much of those hours are spent in 15 to 30-minute dozes or cat naps.

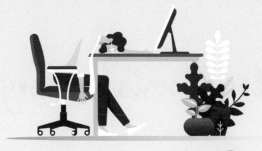

nap-o-pedia

Nano nap

A nano nap of just 10 minutes' light sleep can refresh you and boost your concentration and attention for up to 4 hours.

Power nap

A power nap (about 20 minutes) boosts alertness, memory and information recall, too, with no sleepy hangover.

Happy nap

A happy nap (45 minutes or more) re-establishes your emotional equilibrium by taking you through some REM sleep.

Learning nap

A learning nap (60 to 90 minutes) – or as the Spanish call it, a 'siesta' – gets you some deep sleep, which provides the biggest boost to learning and also motor memory.

How to take a 'coffee' nap (or 'nappaccino')

Use coffee's natural power to wake you up after a planned nap. Drink a cup of coffee immediately before finding yourself a warm, dimly lit and quiet place to lie down. Nod off, and the caffeine will kick in after 15 to 20 minutes. You'll wake up and be raring to go.

How sleep boosts memory

Whether you're trying to learn a new language or study for a big test, there's no need to pull an all-nighter – sleep is the smarter strategy, both before and after learning a new task or new information.

Sleep helps prime your brain to be receptive and alert – ready to learn and acquire new information. After learning, sleep then helps to cement those facts and skills and stop you forgetting them. Memories 'move' from deep within the brain's hippocampus to the higher-level cortex layers – and this transportation happens overnight during sleep.

To be able to learn new things, our brains need to be able to weed out the rubbish and consolidate vital information about what we learned in the day. Luckily, different parts of our brains do this for us while we snooze.

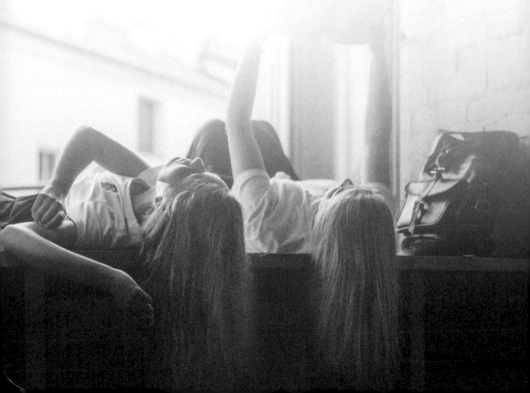

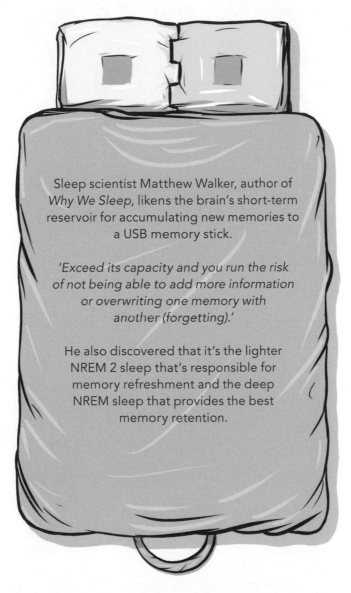

Sleep scientist Matthew Walker, author of *Why We Sleep*, likens the brain's short-term reservoir for accumulating new memories to a USB memory stick.

'Exceed its capacity and you run the risk of not being able to add more information or overwriting one memory with another (forgetting).'

He also discovered that it's the lighter NREM 2 sleep that's responsible for memory refreshment and the deep NREM sleep that provides the best memory retention.

Napping after learning new information outstripped cramming or relaxing with a movie in one study. When tested a week later, the nappers still scored highest.

Some sleepy lit

Writers have always been interested in the world of sleep. Here are a few famously drowsy characters from their pages.

Sleeping Beauty
In the fairy tale popularized by the Brothers Grimm, the parents of a princess are told their daughter will die when she pricks her finger. They rid their kingdom of sharp objects, but in vain. The princess pricks her finger, but instead of dying she falls into a deep enchanted sleep. She is eventually awoken by the kiss of a handsome prince.

The Dormouse in
Alice's Adventures in Wonderland
In Lewis Carroll's *Alice's Adventures in Wonderland*, the Dormouse is always falling asleep. This keeps him out of most of the Tea Party conversations and the other characters frequently poke him. The Mad Hatter even pours hot tea on his nose in a bid to wake him up!

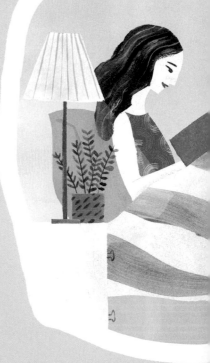

Rip van Winkle
In Washington Irving's eponymous short story, Dutch–American settler Rip van Winkle drinks a strange liquor and sleeps for 20 years. He wakes with a long beard, having slept through the American Revolution, and finds a country he no longer recognizes.

Ebenezer Scrooge in *A Christmas Carol*

In Charles Dickens's *A Christmas Carol*, the miserly Ebenezer Scrooge is trying to sleep on Christmas Eve when he is visited by the ghosts of his former business partner and the spirits of Christmas Past, Present and Yet to Come. Through these apparitions he wakes up full of generosity, having learned the true spirit of Christmas.

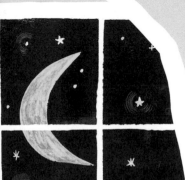

Sarah in *The House of Sleep*

In Jonathan Coe's novel *The House of Sleep*, Sarah is a narcoleptic and Terry is an insomniac. The plot centres on a sleep clinic, where the crazed Dr Dudden sees sleep as a disease that must be eradicated.

Joe in *The Pickwick Papers*

Obesity Hypoventilation Syndrome (OHS), a condition related to sleep apnoea, was first called Pickwickian Syndrome. It's named after Joe, the 'fat boy' in *The Pickwick Papers* by Charles Dickens. Joe has the symptoms of the condition, such as falling asleep in the middle of tasks.

Bertie Wooster

Bertie is a famous late riser in P. G. Wodehouse's Jeeves and Wooster books. When woken early by Jeeves, Bertie asks: 'Ten past nine: is the building on fire?'

Sleep In The Movies

Films have tackled all aspects of sleeping, from late rising to dreams and hibernation. Here are just a few of them:

Four Weddings and a Funeral (1994)
Richard Curtis's comedy famously begins with Hugh Grant lying in bed and discovering that he has overslept and is late for a wedding, followed by a string of expletives.

The Wizard of Oz (1939)
Were the Scarecrow, the Tin Man and the Cowardly Lion all a dream? At the end of the movie Dorothy clicks her heels three times and wakes in her Kansas bedroom with her dog Toto, family and friends, who dismiss her adventures as a dream.

Groundhog Day (1993)
Every day TV weatherman Phil Connors (played by Bill Murray) wakes at his bed and breakfast hotel to hear Sonny and Cher's 'I Got You Babe' on his alarm radio. He keeps waking up to the same song and discovers that every day is Groundhog Day.

The Matrix (1999)
Computer programmer Thomas Anderson (Keanu Reeves) discovers that after a war with artificial intelligence all humans are kept in pods in a sleep-like state and fed a virtual reality view of the world.

2001: A Space Odyssey (1968)

Stanley Kubrick's classic film, adapted from Arthur C. Clarke's novel, features astronauts in suspended animation on board *Discovery One*, bound for Jupiter. Rogue computer HAL turns off the life support systems of three astronauts in suspended animation as Bowman fights to deactivate HAL.

Eternal Sunshine of the Spotless Mind (2004)

Jim Carrey and Kate Winslet star as two former lovers who have both paid a company to erase all memories of each other after their break-up – a process that took place while they were asleep.

Passengers (2016)

Jennifer Lawrence and Chris Pratt play two passengers on a sleeper ship carrying 5,000 colonists to a distant planet. Only they are awakened from an induced hibernation 90 years too early . . .

My Own Private Idaho (1991)

River Phoenix plays Mike, a street hustler with narcolepsy. He has several narcoleptic episodes in the film and in the final scene, after falling into another narcoleptic slumber by the highway, he has his backpack and shoes stolen.

Inception (2010)

Leonardo DiCaprio stars as a thief performing corporate espionage through dream-sharing technology. He infiltrates the subconscious minds of his victims and plants ideas in people's dreams. The film features a three-way shared dream where dying might see them trapped in a subconscious dream world.

Why is yawning so contagious?

For millennia scientists have been puzzled by the function of the yawn. Why do we have this curious behaviour? Is it to release 'noxious air', as Hippocrates once suggested? Or to rebalance gases in the blood, as scientists of the nineteenth century proposed?

Generally, we yawn when we're tired, bored, have a temperature or if we see another person yawning. Once it starts, the urge to yawn cannot be interrupted, however much you try to quash it. It has to proceed all the way to the open-mouthed pose with its long inhalation followed by slow exhalation.

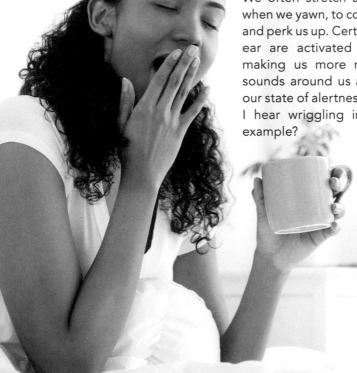

There are several theories about the exact function of yawning – it increases alertness, cools the brain or signals to others our state of vigilance.

We often stretch and fidget about when we yawn, to counter drowsiness and perk us up. Certain muscles in the ear are activated during a yawn, making us more receptive to the sounds around us and feeding into our state of alertness – is that a snake I hear wriggling in the grass, for example?

Some researchers have suggested that yawning brings on a brain chill to stop it overheating. And, indeed, studies show that if you hold a cool compress to your forehead the urge to yawn is drastically reduced.

Because of its contagious or infectious nature – just thinking about yawning can sometimes elicit a yawn – some scientists have suggested that yawning may be a visible signal within a social group. This primitive form of communication shows that one person is sleepy so another may need to step up and take over sentry duty, for instance. Others have suggested it relates to empathy. The jury's still out.

You might well be feeling that irrepressible urge to yawn yourself now, after a few minutes of reading about yawning. If you do, don't try to stifle it, just let it go and enjoy this mysterious but universal action.

50 per cent of people who watch someone yawn will yawn in response. In fact, hearing or even reading about yawning is enough to trigger a yawn.

Athletes often yawn before a race. Cortisol, the stress hormone, is known to trigger yawning.

We yawn before we're even born. Foetuses yawn spontaneously in the womb.

How Sex Makes You Sleepy

Sex and sleep – the perfect duo: sleep boosts your sex drive and regular sex helps you fall asleep more effortlessly. What's not to like? Given that sex also conditions the heart (it's exercise after all), lowers blood pressure, is a stress buster and boosts a sense of wellbeing, it's good to know you're benefiting in all kinds of ways.

Benefits aside, have you ever wondered why some partners seem to fall asleep immediately after orgasm? Apart from sex often taking place in the ideal sleep environment of a dark and cool bedroom on a comfy mattress (we're generalizing here), the brain and body are bathed in a cocktail of chemicals and hormones that serve to calm the mind and relax the body.

Sex and sleep alo

Sex boosts the 'love hormone' **oxytocin** and suppresses the production of the stress hormone **cortisol**. We cuddle up, worries vanish, we relax and then more easily slip into a slumber afterwards. Orgasm, too, floods the brain with multiple chemicals – including **prolactin** (which makes you feel relaxed and sleepy), **endorphins** (the 'feel good' neurotransmitters) and **vasopressin** (which stops you needing the loo at night and is associated with sleep) – which act as a sedative.

Men and women sometimes react differently to the chemical triggers of sex and orgasm. While women may take longer to fall asleep, their sleep is profoundly restful, with enhanced REM sleep.

Fact is, everyone has better sleep after sex, so if you're not getting enough sleep or are finding it hard to drift off, you know what to do.

make me conscious
that I am mortal

– Alexander the Great

The pillow – the past, the now, the future

Today you can select from a cornucopia of pillows – those stuffed with feathers or down, those filled with microbeads or buckwheat, and pillows made from foam designed to mould to your head's unique shape. What's more, they come in myriad shapes: from a giant sausage-like body pillow (great for pregnant women) to a triangular wedge pillow (great for propping you up in bed). But pillows weren't always about comfort, as you'll soon discover.

Stone pillows of Ancient Mesopotamia

These pillows weren't designed for comfort but to keep insects from crawling into the mouths or ears of sleepers.

Jade pillows of Ancient China

The Chinese, despite being able to make soft pillows, preferred the idea of hard ones to bring intellect and health; they believed soft pillows stole vitality from the body during sleep. Jade especially was thought to boost intelligence.

7000 BCE   **1046–256 BCE**

3100–30 BCE

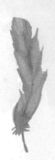

Decorated hard pillows of Ancient Egypt

Made from marble, ivory, ceramic, stone and wood, these carved and decorated pillows with images of the gods were said to ward off bad spirits.

Softer pillows of Ancient Greece and Rome

Finally cloth pillows stuffed with reeds, straw or
feathers arrived; the precursor of the modern-day
pillow was here.

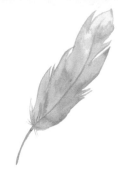

Tall pillows of Japanese Geisha

To avoid messing up their elaborate coiffures,
Geisha had to learn to sleep on a tall pillow, or
taka-makura. Even though this slightly padded rest
(made of wood or porcelain with a bag of straw)
cradled the base of the neck, it probably felt like the
stone pillows of old.

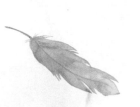

785 BCE–1453 AD   1760–1840 AD

500–1500 AD

European Middle Ages straw pillows

Now becoming more widespread, these pillows
had to be re-stuffed regularly to deal with mouse
and mould damage.

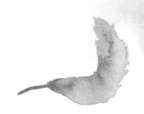

The ubiquitous soft pillow

With the advent of technology in the Industrial Revolution, soft pillows were mass-produced for the first time.

Smart sleep pillows

Some are height-adjustable so you can tweak to your perfect support level; some can play music and track your movement at night with sensors; other pillows – with listening microphones and pumps and motors, albeit small ones – give you a gentle nudge if you snore; yet others offer a thermoregulated sleeping experience, since a cool pillow helps you fall asleep. There's even a robot pillow that synchronizes your breathing to its breathing to relax you ready for slumber, or one that plays a soundtrack of a heartbeat.

1750–1840 AD

2018

1990s

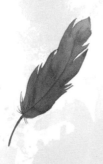

Space-age foam pillows

With the invention of memory foam by NASA in the 1970s, it wasn't too long before it found its way to the bedroom.

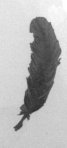

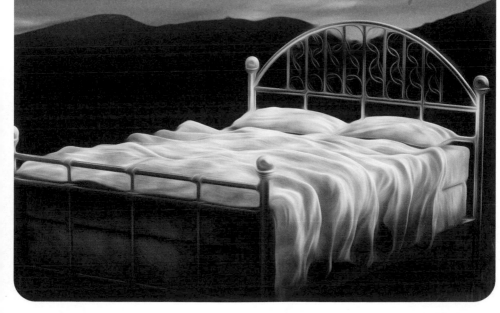

Source: A bedroom poll
from National Sleep
Foundation/US

41%

31%

15%

<1%

9%

4%

USED NO
PILLOWS

USED ONE
PILLOW

USED TWO
PILLOWS

USED THREE
PILLOWS

USED FOUR
PILLOWS

USED FIVE
PILLOWS

A Bedroom Poll

Sleep

Problems

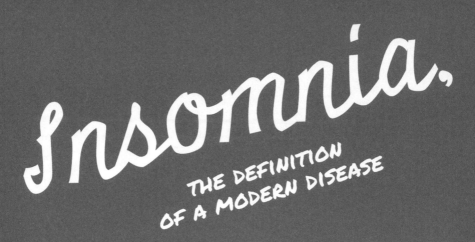

Insomnia,

THE DEFINITION OF A MODERN DISEASE

Insomnia

mass noun: in-som-ni-a

Habitual sleeplessness; inability to sleep.

Origin early seventeenth century: from Latin, from *insomnis* 'sleepless', from *in-* (expressing negation) + *somnus* 'sleep'.

A modern, busy life comes with the odd night of broken sleep or a mind buzzing with 'what if?'s for the next day to keep you awake. But this temporary tiredness is not insomnia.

Doctors diagnose insomnia if you're regularly having trouble falling asleep or trouble staying asleep. And by 'regularly' they mean 3 nights a week for a period of 3 months.

The Great British Bedtime Report showed that almost half of Britons say that stress or worry keeps them awake at night.

The two most common factors behind insomnia are worry and anxiety. These emotional conditions work against everything your body naturally wants and needs for sleep. They:

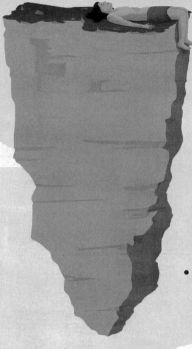

- Activate the 'fight or flight' response, which sees stress hormones surging around the body (when what's needed for sleep is relaxation not alertness).

- Raise metabolism, which in turn raises core body temperature (which needs to dip so you can nod off).

- Promote activity in the emotion-generating regions of the brain (when these need to power down for initial sleep).

Other causes of insomnia are bad sleeping habits and medicines.

And to add insult to injury, the sleep that insomniacs eventually do get is not refreshing: their deep NREM sleep is less powerful and their REM sleep is fragmented.

Struggling to find the snooze button? Waking up with the dawn chorus? Then turn over the page to discover 10 tips for a good night's sleep, including creating the right environment, the importance of a regular sleep schedule, how to deal with those niggling worries and ways of unwinding from the day.

10 steps to a good night's sleep

Sometimes referred to as sleep hygiene, these small steps can make the world of difference to your sleep experience.

1 Your sleep schedule

Go to bed and wake up at consistent times every day, including weekends. If you ever take a nap don't do it after 3 p.m.

2 Get outside every day

Expose yourself to plenty of daylight in the day to help tweak your body's inbuilt clock for sleep.

3 Cool down

Take an evening bath (it'll make you feel toasty but actually helps lower your core body temperature) and dial down the radiators in your bedroom to between 16°C and 18°C.

4 Get physical

Regular exercise literally does tire you out but leaving it until late in the evening has the reverse effect; don't exercise within 3 hours of your bedtime.

5 Check your caffeine intake

Caffeine can interfere with your body's natural sleepiness; if you're sensitive to its effects, avoid caffeine-containing drinks and chocolate.

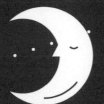

6

Dim the lights

Avoid bright lights in the evenings, especially the blue light of LED devices, to help your body listen to its melatonin sleep trigger.

7 Let go of worries

A bedside duo of pen and notebook allows you to write down worries or urgent to-dos, so you can unwind and focus on falling asleep instead of fretting about tomorrow.

8

Skip the nightcap

Skip the nightcap – alcohol before bed disrupts your deep sleep, so you'll wake up feeling unrefreshed.

9

Schedule screen-free time

If you need to check your email one last time or quickly catch up on social media, make sure the last time you look at your phone is 1 to 2 hours before your bedtime; keep those last hours before sleep sacrosanct.

And relax 10

Find what works for you to de-stress, be it meditation, breathing exercises, podcasts, a Sleep Story or just settling down with a good book.

Scent-sational Sleep Solutions

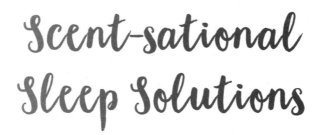

Essential oils are the potent, distilled forms of all kinds of flowers.* Such botanical scents have long been known for their natural beneficial powers – for relaxing you (rose, geranium or jasmine) or pepping you up (eucalyptus or menthol), for instance. But there is another well-known essential oil, with its long-loved calming qualities, which can help your body relax and a buzzing mind unwind, ready for sleep to arrive: lavender.

*Be careful about applying anything directly to skin and avoid using around anyone with epilepsy or high blood pressure.

Let master storyteller Stephen Fry take you on a calming journey through the lavender fields of Provence. Don't forget to inhale deeply.

'You'll smell it before you even see it. That unmistakable aroma that fills your nose and seeps into your senses, instantly mellowing into a smooth and soothing scent. You breathe deeply, inhaling and exhaling this floral cloud and, as you do, something unexplained washes over you. Slowly at first you feel your body begin to release its pent-up tension. Your breath becomes deeper, deliberate, calm. Inexplicably those deep lines in your furrowed brow one by one unfurl as you slowly, and gently, begin to relax. The scent is lavender.'

Stephen Fry
Blue Gold

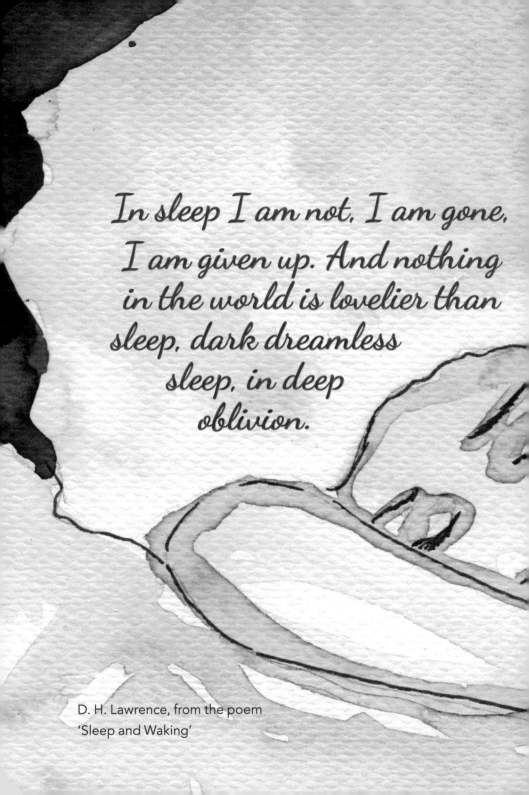

In sleep I am not, I am gone, I am given up. And nothing in the world is lovelier than sleep, dark dreamless sleep, in deep oblivion.

D. H. Lawrence, from the poem 'Sleep and Waking'

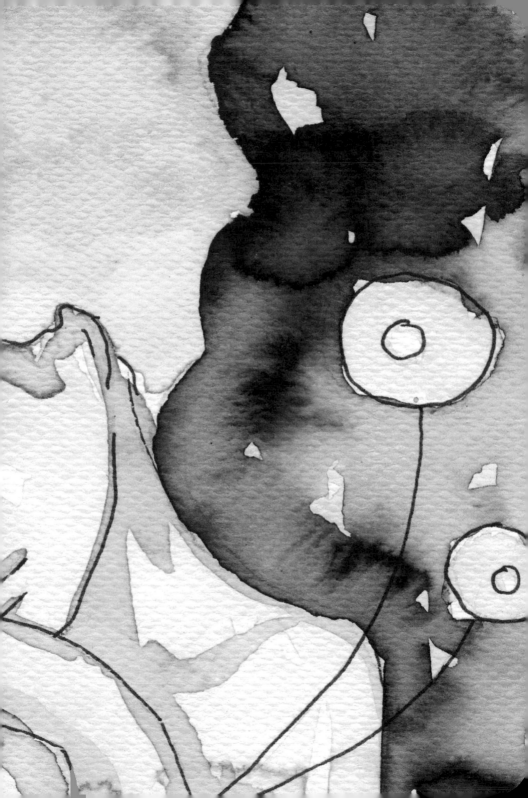

Cures for insomnia

Simon Cowell turned to hypnotist Paul McKenna, Jennifer Aniston took heed from Arianna Huffington, and Kim Cattrall tried CBT to cure insomnia. Apart from setting good sleeping habits and dealing with worries, what other 'cures' exist for insomniacs?

CBT

Cognitive behavioural therapy – or CBT for short – can change any unhelpful thoughts or behaviours that are causing your insomnia. There are various approaches of CBT designed to deal with insomnia, including:

Sleep restriction – it sounds counter-intuitive, but this programme limits your sleep so that you become increasingly tired (a planned mild sleep deprivation) and avoids the lying-in-bed-awake scenario that can become a habit. Sleep time increases once your sleep improves.

Stimulus control – this strategy helps to build an association between the bedroom and sleep by allowing only certain activities in the bedroom (sleep and sex); it may come with set bedtimes and wake times too.

Relaxation training – whether you follow a 2-minute heart-slowing feature on your activity tracker or listen to a guided meditation, calming your body and mind can create the right conditions for sleep.

Hypnotism or hypnotherapy

Whether you use this technique for relaxation purposes or to plant the suggestion of better sleep deep within your mind, it can show results in only a few sessions. You'll be taken into a trance-like state and follow verbal cues from the therapist; some people even fall asleep during a session. And no swinging watches, guaranteed.

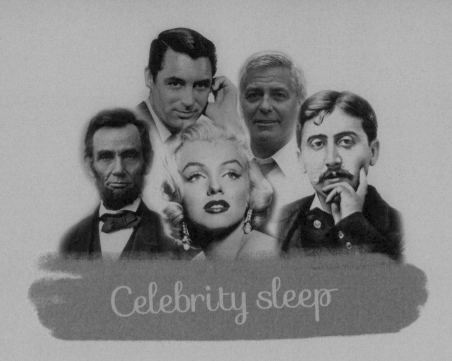

Celebrity sleep

Insomnia doesn't discriminate and can ravage any person's sleep, famous or not. Celebrities are not immune from niggles that keep them up at night; in fact, often their work schedules don't naturally align with all that we know helps a good night's sleep.

Famous insomniacs:

Abraham Lincoln
Arianna Huffington
Bill Clinton
Cary Grant
George Clooney
Heath Ledger
Jimi Hendrix
Lady Gaga

Madonna
Marcel Proust
Marilyn Monroe
Napoleon Bonaparte
Prince
Rihanna
Simon Cowell
Vincent Van Gogh

Only 1.5 per cent of the Hadza people in Tanzania and 2.5 per cent of the San people in Namibia say they regularly have problems falling or staying asleep. Neither group has a word for insomnia in their language.

A RUFFLED MIND MAKES A RESTLESS PILLOW

CHARLOTTE BRONTË,
THE PROFESSOR

Sleep inequalities

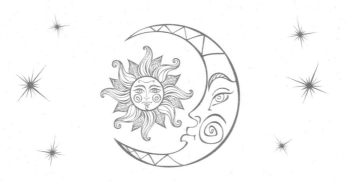

Fact:

Women report sleeping badly more than men – insomnia is almost twice as common in women as in men. Whether this reflects men's reluctance to disclose such personal information is hard to know. What is known is that a woman's hormonal cycle is linked to sleep disruptions.

Six reasons that women sleep worse than men:

- Greater fluctuations in hormones (oestrogen and progesterone), causing discomfort and changes in body temperature.

- Anxiety and depression are twice as common in women.

- Pregnancy and its associated night-time discomfort.

- More responsibility for newborns and young children.

- Restless leg syndrome – women suffer more.

- The menopause brings more hormone fluctuations, hot flushes and night sweats.

Source: *Sunday Times*

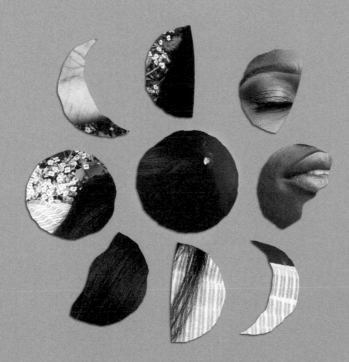

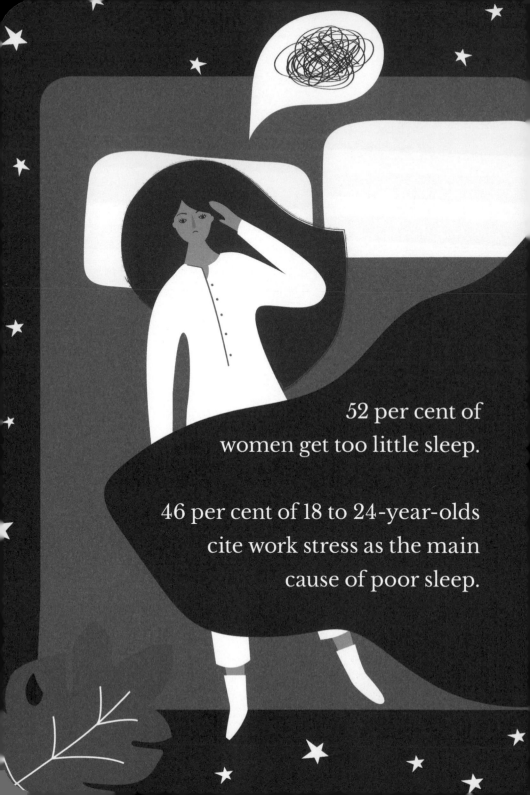

52 per cent of women get too little sleep.

46 per cent of 18 to 24-year-olds cite work stress as the main cause of poor sleep.

59 per cent of women aged 65 or over enjoy good or very good sleep.

Women are 40 per cent more likely than men 'always' to sleep badly, reveals a survey of 4,279 Britons and Americans, conducted by pollsters YouGov, on behalf of Calm.

Why are men always hot and women cold?

A common scenario the world over – a man lies in bed with the duvet thrown off while his partner is snuggled under the covers dreaming of cashmere bedsocks. When it's freezing outside, it's great to have a human hot water bottle to snuggle up to in bed, but when it's summer such a warm partner can sap any chances of sleep. There are biological reasons behind the temperature differences – based on body size, metabolism and hormones. Perhaps the Scandinavians have got it right, with their two-duvet approach.

The Best
and wo

As a recent YouGov poll commissioned by Calm found, Sunday may be the day of rest but it seems the night of restlessness. Three times as many of us sleep badly on Sunday as on any other single night, according to a survey of 4,279 Americans and Britons. Thursday, in contrast, seems the true night of rest. The biggest reason that so many people sleep badly on Sundays is that the weekend is when they throw off their normal sleep routine, says Dr Steve Orma, a clinical psychologist and insomnia specialist.

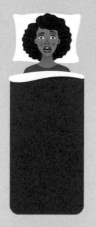 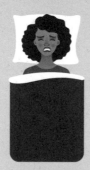 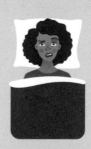 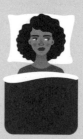

SUNDAY 46% MONDAY 17% SATURDAY 9% WEDNESDAY 9%

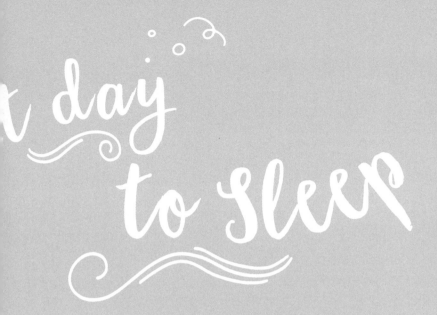

t day
to sleep

Thursday is the night of the week when people report sleeping best. Sunday is by far the opposite, mentioned by almost half of all respondents as the night they sleep worst.

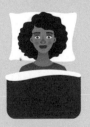

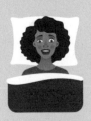

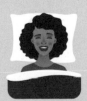

TUESDAY 8%   FRIDAY 7%   THURSDAY 5%

Strange sleeping disorders you've probably never heard of

Sleep walking and talking aren't the only weird goings-on in the night. Discover the array of sleep disorders that range from plain strange to downright terrifying.

Hypnogogic jerks
Have you ever woken yourself with muscle twitches or jumps as you're nodding off? These mysterious jerks are often accompanied by a sense of falling.

Exploding head syndrome
Not quite the terrifying prospect suggested by its name, this actually harmless condition is the sensation of a super-loud noise (like an explosion or a gunshot) just as you're falling asleep. No one's sure what causes it.

Sleep paralysis
Usually your brain switches off your body during REM sleep so that you can't act out your dreams, but sometimes the timing of switching this paralysis off is out of sync, for up to several minutes. Scarily, you wake up but without being able to move or speak; some people report a feeling of being crushed.

REM sleep disorder
The opposite of sleep paralysis, where the brain fails to paralyse the body so a person can act out their dreams – yelling, punching, kicking and jumping out of bed are common.

Kleine–Levin syndrome

Also known as 'sleeping beauty' syndrome since an affected person can sleep for up to 23 hours a day for weeks at a time. In their brief waking moments, sufferers display unusual behaviours, including binge eating, hallucinations and heightened sex drive.

Sleep-related eating disorder

Beans on toast at 3 a.m., anyone? People with this condition can cook and eat while they're asleep and not remember a thing.

The space between breaths

Stressed out about not getting to sleep? Then turn to the ancient practice of yoga and discover the value of taking a pause, using this breath control exercise or *kumbhaka*. It can help you relax, unwind and even tip you into slumber when practised at bedtime.

Simply listening to the natural rhythm of your breath can lull you into a state of profound relaxation – it even slows your heart rate when done purposefully. Do it just before bed to mirror what the body naturally does as it's slipping into sleep and you'll find sleep comes more easily.

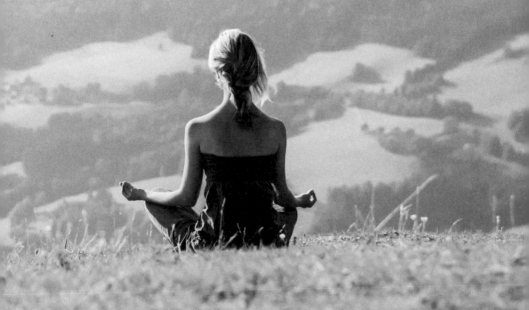

Kumbhaka

Breathe in for a count of 4.

Hold that breath for a count of 4.

Breathe out for a count of 8.

Repeat for up to 30 minutes.

Sleep Idioms

Sleep like a log. Sleep like a baby.

Drop off to sleep. Oversleep.

Sleep tight. Catch some Zs.

Out for the count. Dead to the world.

Light sleeper. **HEAVY SLEEPER**

Burn the candle at both ends.

Sleep on it. Let sleeping dogs lie.

Sleeping partner.

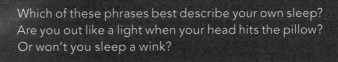

Which of these phrases best describe your own sleep?
Are you out like a light when your head hits the pillow?
Or won't you sleep a wink?

Nod off. Fast asleep. Hit the sack.

Lie in. Cat nap. Forty winks.

Tuck someone in. Get some kip.

Goes out like a light. Turn in.

Barely keep my eyes open.

Pull an all-nighter. Not sleep a wink.

Tossing and turning

Lose sleep over something.

Do you duvet?

Long gone are the days of sheets with hospital corners and heavy blankets. The sixties welcomed the 'continental quilt' to the UK – it was sold by Sir Terence Conran's Habitat with the strapline 'the 10-second bed'.

While tucking someone into bed might have become a thing of the past, the duvet revolutionized bedmaking (just shake and go) and sleeping. No more would you have to be pressed to the bed by the weight of blankets, since a lightweight feather- or synthetic-filled quilt could keep you at just the right temperature.

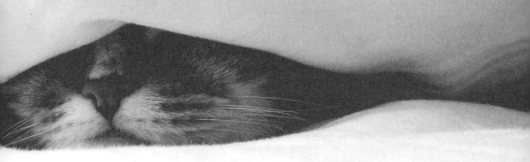

What is your duvet's tog rating?

The Shirley Togmeter (an actual machine to test for tog!) gives a duvet a rating of what's known as its thermal insulance. From a colloquial word for outer garment or coat (from the French *togue* or Latin *toga*), tog is the easier-to-say version of the SI unit m2K/W. The lower the tog number, the cooler the duvet.

Summer duvet	3 to 4.5 tog
Spring/autumn duvet	7.5 to 10.5 tog
Winter duvet	12 to 3.5 tog

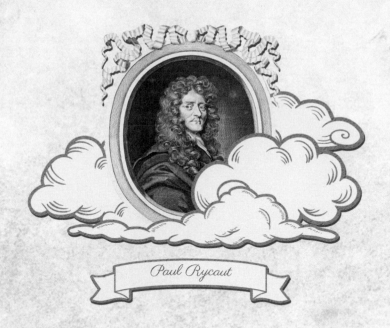

Paul Rycaut

The inventor of the duvet?

As well as writing an illustrated account of lemmings and their migratory habits, Paul Rycaut (1629–1700), a British diplomat, tried to get the idea of eiderdown-stuffed coverings off the ground after sleeping under something similar on a trip to Germany. The cost of the fillings then was perhaps prohibitively expensive to make a saleable duvet and the Brits seemed wedded to their blankets for night-time warmth. He was obviously ahead of his time.

An Icelandic eiderdown duvet could set you back around £10,000.

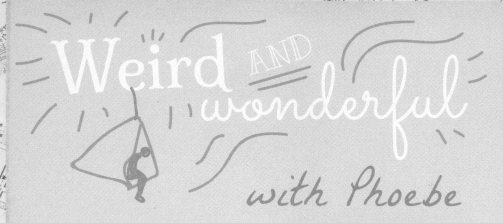

Weird AND wonderful
with Phoebe

Phoebe Smith has slept in some pretty unusual places. The author of wild camping book *Extreme Sleeps*, and Calm's Sleep Storyteller-in-Residence, is the world's only 'extreme sleep adventurer'. Here are some of the strange bedplaces she's ended up in.

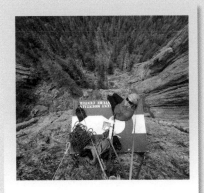

HALFWAY UP A CLIFF

Cliff camping is a scary night's sleep strapped on to a portaledge canvas platform stuck halfway up a massive cliff. Sleepers have to rappel down the sheer rockface first. Smith has tried this in Estes Park, Colorado, USA and the Avon Gorge in Bristol, UK.

UNDER A GIANT BOULDER

Smith enjoys sleeping under the Shelter Stone in the Cairngorms, Scotland. It is a huge boulder with a sunken chamber underneath it, ideal for watching the snow come down outside.

places to sleep,

Smith

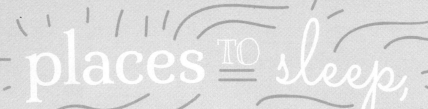

HANGING FROM A TREE
In a Bavarian adventure park she climbed 9 metres up a tree and slept in a combined pup tent and hammock, gently swaying as she slept.

ON A GLACIER
Smith has slept in the Svalbard glacier in Norway, 15 metres inside the ice. She has also slept on the Khumbu glacier near the Everest Base Camp in Nepal.

OVER THE GREAT BARRIER REEF
A pontoon floating over the Great Barrier Reef was her bed for the night after a day snorkelling in the Australian coral wonder.

IN THE WRECK OF A WORLD WAR II BOMBER
Smith spent a night among the decaying wreckage of a World War II American bomber on moorland in Bleaklow, Derbyshire, UK.

IN A HERMIT'S CAVE
She has slept in an English Lake District cave on Castle Crag, where 1930s bearded hermit Millican Dalton lived for many years.

ON A VOLCANO
For a really hot night in bed, Smith slept near mud pools on the crater of the active Telica volcano in Nicaragua, hearing rumblings as she slept.

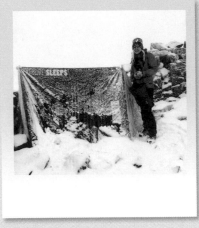

IN THE DESERT
She's slept on a rock ledge in the sandy desert made famous by Lawrence of Arabia in Wadi Rum, Jordan.

IN ANTARCTICA
She's arrived by ship and slept in a tent at the bottom of the world in Antarctica, waking up to find penguins outside her tent door.

IN THE AUSTRALIAN BUSH
Sleeping out under the stars in the 'red centre' of Australia first inspired Smith to pursue her career of wild camping.

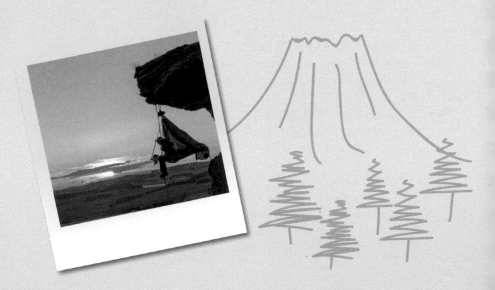

Humans are strange creatures – you name it, they can sleep there.

IN SPACE
The first man to sleep in space was USSR cosmonaut Gherman Titov in 1961, on board *Vostok 2*, which was orbiting the Earth. After securing his floating arms with a belt he reported a very good night's sleep.

ON THE FELLS
The great English fellwalker and guidebook writer Alfred Wainwright would often sleep in the open on the mountains of the Lake District, with only a blanket and pipe as comfort.

IN A COFFIN
A self-proclaimed vampire called Darkness Vlad Tepes revealed in 2016 that he slept in a custom-made coffin. He changed his name by deed poll and sleeps in his coffin in Blackburn, Lancashire, UK.

IN A TRANSPARENT BEDROOM ON A CLIFF
In Peru, one adventure company has transparent capsules hanging off a sheer rockface on a 3,650m mountain, reached via a zipline ferrata climb. The suites have bedrooms, dining rooms and a bathroom for a luxury night of high living.

IN A CRANE
A hotel in the Netherlands offers nights in the cabin of a disused Docklands crane. Breakfast is delivered by the internal lift.

IN AN ICE HOTEL
In Sweden, the Ice Hotel in Jukkasjärvi is made from ice in the River Torne. Bedrooms are a chilly –5°C. Snowsuits are provided.

10 WEIRDEST-EVER *Insomnia* CURES

Throughout history a lack of sleep has promoted desperate insomniacs to try a wide variety of different remedies. Here are some of the more unusual ones, from a YouGov survey for Calm.

1 Dormouse FAT

rubbed on the soles of your feet (dates back to the Romans; resurfaced in Elizabethan England)

2 FRIED *lettuce*

(a traditional French folk remedy)

3 SEA slug ENTRAILS

eaten before bed
(a traditional Japanese
folk remedy)

4 DOG'S earwax

rubbed on your teeth
(recommended in Renaissance Italy)

5 BILE OF castrated BOAR

drunk in a potion (all the rage in the
Middle Ages, apparently, when it
was also used as an anaesthetic)

6 POINTING your BED northward

(Charles Dickens swore by it)

7 Yellow Soap

lathered in your hair (in Victorian
Britain, you lathered your head
with yellow soap, then tied your
hair in a napkin – naturally!)

8 Lettuce OPIUM

(extracted from wild lettuce
stems and drunk in a brew
by the ancient Egyptians)

9 CINNAMON banana tea

(advocated by some today as a natural sleep aid)

10 CURLING & UNCURLING YOUR TOES

(a relaxation exercise that
doubles as a sleepiness prompt)

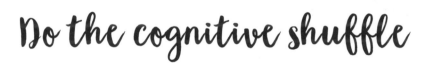

Do the cognitive shuffle

Trick yourself to sleep

If that all-elusive shut-eye is nowhere to be found, perhaps this trick called cognitive shuffling, designed by Canadian cognitive scientist Luc Beaudoin, could help.

The technique gets you to imagine random objects but without making any connections between them, to lull the brain into a pre-sleep grogginess so it's primed for slumber. Such visualization can quieten your mind and help you doze off.

1. Get comfy in bed.

2. Pick a letter at random. Visualize a word starting with that letter (five letters long or more); it needs to be an emotionally neutral word. So, for example, 'O' for 'ocean' – imagine sitting on a beach staring at the vast expanse of water. Imagine the scene but don't start making up a story or scenario. Next, think of another word starting with 'O' – orangutan, olive, oatmeal . . .

3. Once you've exhausted the 'O' list, it's time to work through 'C' then 'E' then 'A' then 'N' – if you get that far. Some people nod off within a few minutes while others take up to 20 minutes before drifting off to dreamland.

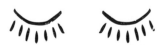

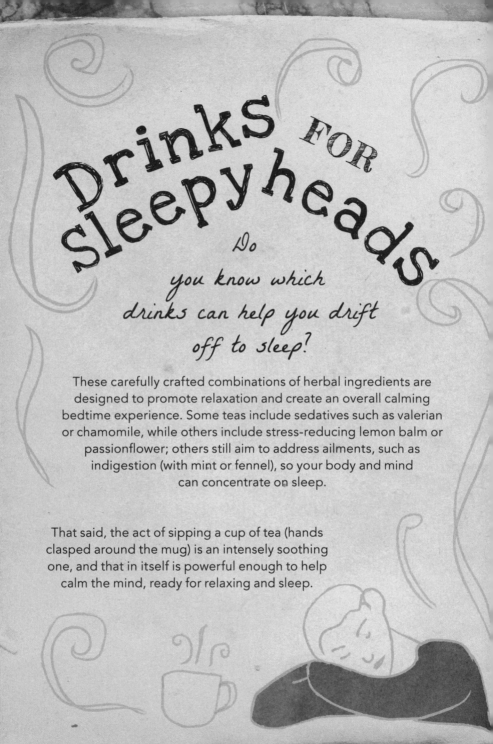

Drinks FOR Sleepyheads

Do you know which drinks can help you drift off to sleep?

These carefully crafted combinations of herbal ingredients are designed to promote relaxation and create an overall calming bedtime experience. Some teas include sedatives such as valerian or chamomile, while others include stress-reducing lemon balm or passionflower; others still aim to address ailments, such as indigestion (with mint or fennel), so your body and mind can concentrate on sleep.

That said, the act of sipping a cup of tea (hands clasped around the mug) is an intensely soothing one, and that in itself is powerful enough to help calm the mind, ready for relaxing and sleep.

Chamomile tea

Scientists are still trying to isolate which of chamomile's many components are responsible for its calming and sedative powers, but its effects have been known for centuries. Allow your chamomile flowers to steep for up to 10 minutes for maximum flavour and effect, and enjoy 30 minutes before bedtime. Always check with your GP before serving these drinks to a small child, or a vulnerable or pregnant person.

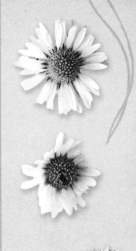

Top bedtime teas

- Chamomile
- Fennel (great for colicky babies)
- Valerian
- Lemon balm
- Passionflower
- Lemongrass

- Ginger
- Mint
- Red teas with rosehips and hibiscus
- Honeybush
- Rooibos
- Tulsi (a type of basil)

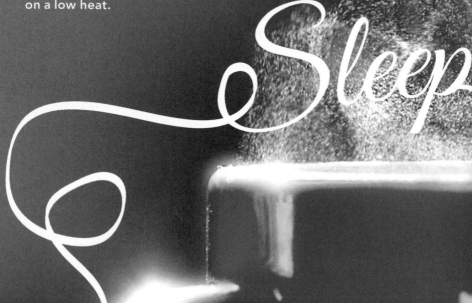

Golden Milk

This spiced draught, with beneficial curcumin from the turmeric, protects against the effects of sleep deprivation. Double up if you want to make it for two.

- **240ml of your favourite milk**
- **½ tsp ground turmeric**
- **¼ tsp ground cinnamon**
- **A small pinch of ground black pepper**
- **A small pinch of ground ginger**
- **Cayenne pepper (optional; if you like a kick of heat)**
- **½ tsp of your favourite sweetener**

Simply blend all the ingredients together in a food processor and then warm through in a saucepan on a low heat.

Sleep

Malted milk

With its combination of warm milk and nostalgic maltiness (not to mention a blend of magnesium, vitamin B, iron, zinc and phosphorus), this old-fashioned favourite will relax you and make you feel drowsy.

Sour cherry juice

The sleep-promoting hormone melatonin is naturally present in foods, including tart cherries, goji berries and raspberries. Research has shown significant but modest improvements in sleep after boosting melatonin levels with two doses a day of this super-tasty juice.

drinks

The comfort of Cl

It's no coincidence that laundry product manufacturers try to sell you never-ending freshness in their TV ads, since it turns out that 73 per cent of people say that they sleep better on fresh sheets, according to a 2012 study by the US's National Sleep Foundation. Whether you like to iron out every wrinkle on bedsheets (therapeutic for some), just shake the duvet and go, or love to plump up a stack of pillows, the experience of lying back and relaxing on just-washed sheets or a just-changed bed seems to have soporific qualities for many.

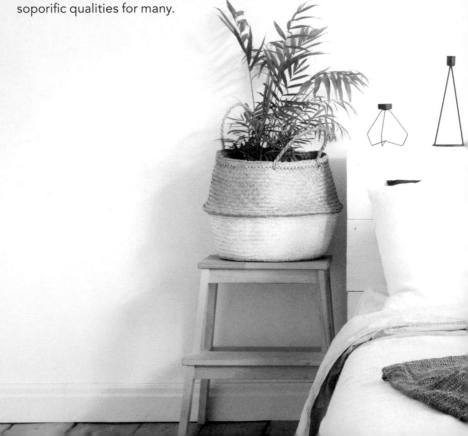

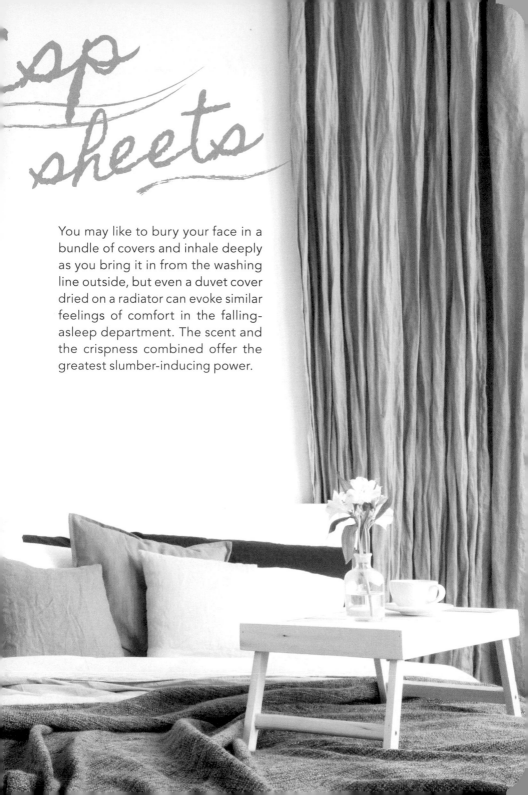

crisp sheets

You may like to bury your face in a bundle of covers and inhale deeply as you bring it in from the washing line outside, but even a duvet cover dried on a radiator can evoke similar feelings of comfort in the falling-asleep department. The scent and the crispness combined offer the greatest slumber-inducing power.

Complete in the morning

Start date: __/__/__ Day of week:	Day 1	Day 2	Day 3	Day 4	Day 5	Day 6	Day 7
I went to bed last night at:	PM/AM	PM/AM	PM/AM	PM/AM	PM/AM	PM/AM	PM/AM
I got out of bed this morning at:	AM/PM	AM/PM	AM/PM	AM/PM	AM/PM	AM/PM	AM/PM

Last night I fell asleep:

	Day 1	Day 2	Day 3	Day 4	Day 5	Day 6	Day 7
Easily	☐	☐	☐	☐	☐	☐	☐
After some time	☐	☐	☐	☐	☐	☐	☐
With difficulty	☐	☐	☐	☐	☐	☐	☐

I woke up during the night:

	Day 1	Day 2	Day 3	Day 4	Day 5	Day 6	Day 7
# of times							
# of minutes							

Last night I slept a total of:

My sleep was disturbed by:

List mental or physical factors including noise, lights, pets, allergies, temperature, discomfort, stress, etc.

When I woke up for the day, I felt:

	Day 1	Day 2	Day 3	Day 4	Day 5	Day 6	Day 7
Refreshed	☐	☐	☐	☐	☐	☐	☐
Somewhat refreshed	☐	☐	☐	☐	☐	☐	☐
Fatigued	☐	☐	☐	☐	☐	☐	☐

Notes:
Record any other factors that may affect your sleep (i.e. hours of work shift or monthly cycle for women)

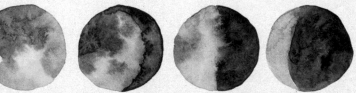

Complete at the end of day

Day of the week:	Day 1	Day 2	Day 3	Day 4	Day 5	Day 6	Day 7

I consumed caffeinated drinks in the: (M)orning, (A)fternoon, (E)vening, (N/A)

M / A / E / NA							

I exercised for at least 20 minutes in the: (M)orning, (A)fternoon, (E)vening, (N/A)

Medications I took today:

Took a nap? (Circle one) If yes, for how long?	Yes No	Yes No	Yes No	Yes No	Yes No	Yes No	Yes No

During the day, how likely was I to doze off while performing daily activities:

No chance, slight chance, moderate chance, high chance

Throughout the day, my mood was ... Very pleasant, pleasant, unpleasant, very unpleasant

Approximately 2–3 hours before going to bed, I consumed:

	Day 1	Day 2	Day 3	Day 4	Day 5	Day 6	Day 7
Alcohol	☐	☐	☐	☐	☐	☐	☐
A heavy meal	☐	☐	☐	☐	☐	☐	☐
Caffeine	☐	☐	☐	☐	☐	☐	☐
Not applicable	☐	☐	☐	☐	☐	☐	☐

In the hour before going to sleep, my bedtime routine included:

List activities including reading a book, using electronics, taking a bath, doing relaxation exercises, etc.

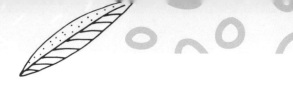
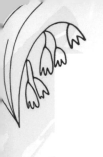

WHAT'S MESSING
with your sleep?

The quality of your slumber as well as how much shut-eye you get depends on many factors, other than those inbuilt biological ones. Luckily this means you can do something about them to steer your bedtime hours towards sleep, not sleeplessness.

- [ ] *Watching TV before bed*
- [ ] *Scrolling through social media*
- [ ] *Bright lighting*
- [ ] *Eating chocolate late in the day*
- [ ] *Checking and/or answering emails before bed*
- [ ] *Night-time parenting or caregiving*
- [ ] *Not making enough time for relaxation*
- [ ] *Staying out late*
- [ ] *Drinking coffee or other high-caffeine beverages after a certain time of day*

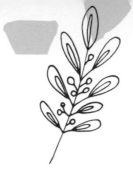

HOW MANY OF THESE
apply to you?

- [ ] Late-night gym sessions
- [ ] A hot bedroom
- [ ] Inconsistent sleeping hours
- [ ] Noise during sleep hours
- [ ] Eating close to bedtime
- [ ] Stress
- [ ] Drinking alcohol in the evening
- [ ] Sleeping in at the weekends
- [ ] A busy mind

Sleep like a Scandinavian

Bedtime tussles over the duvet be gone! Follow the Scandinavian style of sleeping with two duvets – rather than one – for better sleep and more harmony in the bedroom.

Anyone who's been gripped by *The Bridge* or other Scandi-noir TV series may well have noticed oddities in the bedroom backdrops. Two single duvets on a double bed, rather than one. What's going on?

It's common for each sleeper to get their own duvet in countries such as Sweden, Denmark, Norway and Finland. There's always possibilities for cuddling, but when it comes to the serious business of sleep, you can cosy down, *hygge*-style, and never have to worry about waking up chilly as your partner has rolled themselves up with the duvet, leaving you out in the cold. Such supreme comfort means superb sleep, all round.

Couples who sleep together have their sleep interrupted 50 per cent more than those who sleep solo.

1 in 7 British couples sleeps in separate beds.

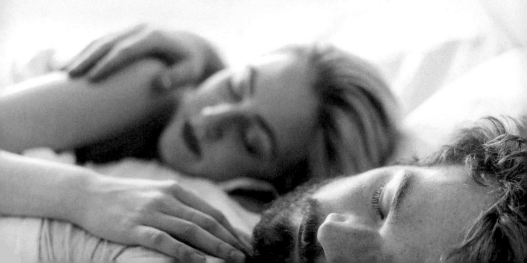

Open that window!

While a lower body temperature is a crucial trigger for slumber, an open window does more than bring in cooler air from outside – it also gives a better balance of carbon dioxide (CO_2) in the bedroom. A study at Eindhoven University in the Netherlands showed that lower levels of CO_2 were tied to better-quality sleep and fewer night-time awakenings.

Design your bedroom

Give yourself the best chance of a good night's sleep by tweaking your bedroom environment. Just a few adjustments can make all the difference to the quantity and quality of your shut-eye.

- Dial down the temperature or open a window. A drop in core body temperature is vital on the route to snooze.

- Green up your space. Plants can help improve your sleep environment by oxygenating the air, removing air pollutants and improving humidity. Green ivy and aloe vera are great, but any house plant in the bedroom can improve mood and reduce stress.

The spider plant grows super quickly (it produces little 'babies' you can give to your friends) and can remove up to 90 per cent of the toxins from the air in your bedroom in just 2 days.

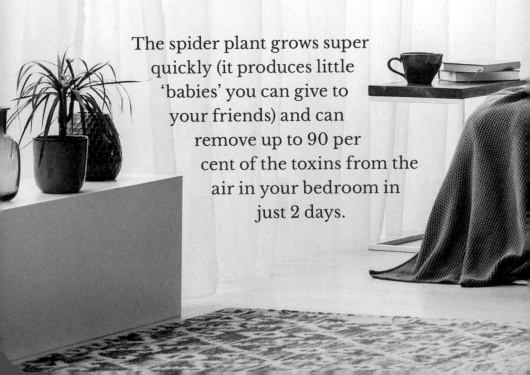

with sleep in mind

- Paint one wall blue or add accents of blue around the room on curtains or bedding. Soft blues have a low saturation and are seen by the brain as mentally soothing and calming.

- Block out the light with blackout curtains or blinds (or wear an eye mask) to reinforce to your brain and body that it's dark and time to sleep. It also helps to keep out the early light of summer mornings.

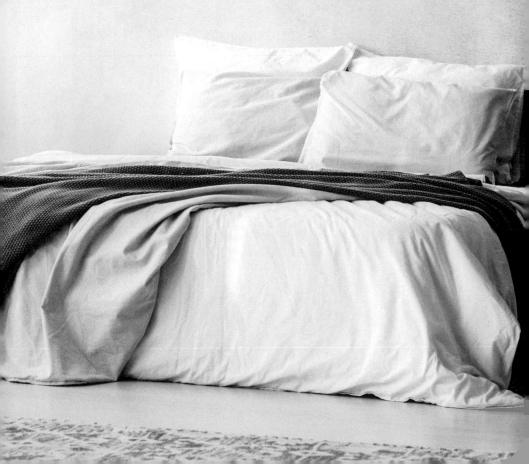

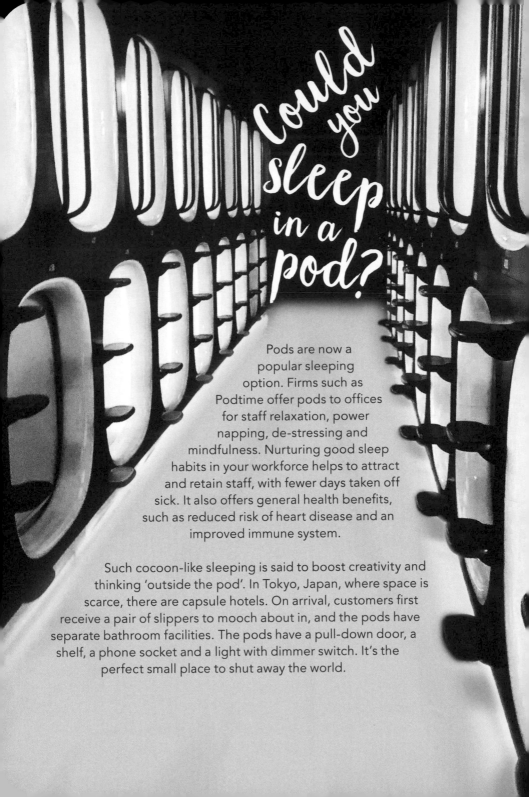

Could you sleep in a pod?

Pods are now a popular sleeping option. Firms such as Podtime offer pods to offices for staff relaxation, power napping, de-stressing and mindfulness. Nurturing good sleep habits in your workforce helps to attract and retain staff, with fewer days taken off sick. It also offers general health benefits, such as reduced risk of heart disease and an improved immune system.

Such cocoon-like sleeping is said to boost creativity and thinking 'outside the pod'. In Tokyo, Japan, where space is scarce, there are capsule hotels. On arrival, customers first receive a pair of slippers to mooch about in, and the pods have separate bathroom facilities. The pods have a pull-down door, a shelf, a phone socket and a light with dimmer switch. It's the perfect small place to shut away the world.

Why don't adults fall out of bed?

Even when adults are asleep, certain senses remain active. The **proprioceptive system** (your sensory receptor) operates all the time, even during sleep, relying on nerve endings to transmit data to the brain about where the body is in relation to the environment. The same system helps us stand upright and is the reason people can walk in their sleep.

Every change of position through the night is relayed to the brain. Through these receptors we avoid bedtime calamities, such as rolling out of bed. The sensory systems of young children are not so well developed, which is why they might occasionally fall out of bed.

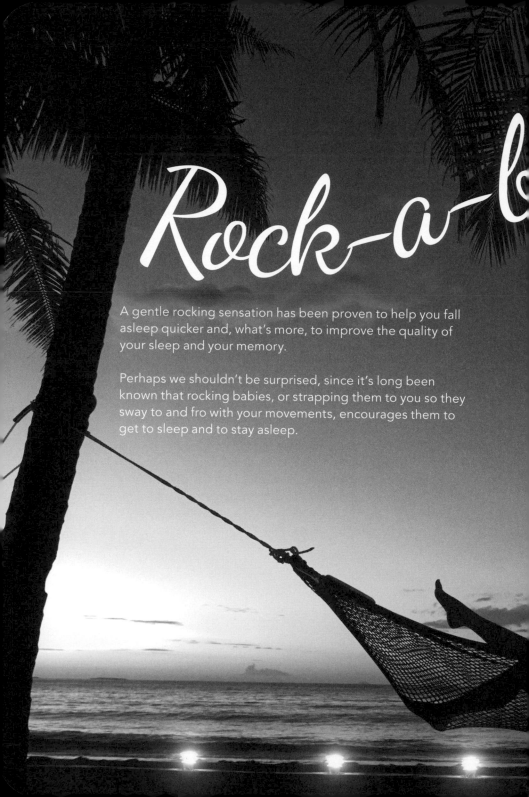

Rock-a-b

A gentle rocking sensation has been proven to help you fall asleep quicker and, what's more, to improve the quality of your sleep and your memory.

Perhaps we shouldn't be surprised, since it's long been known that rocking babies, or strapping them to you so they sway to and fro with your movements, encourages them to get to sleep and to stay asleep.

ge baby

High-tech rocking beds may already be in development, but the low-tech solution of a hammock would work just as well for anyone suffering with insomnia. Despite only 18 people being involved in one study the results were significant – a shorter transition to sleep, longer ultra-deep sleep and better results on a memory test.

And the award goes to . .

Fancy your chances at a record-breaking sleep event? Find out what prizes and records have been awarded in the world of sleep.

Guinness World Records now has a policy against recording or publishing records about how long a person can go without sleep, as it's so potentially dangerous for mind and body.

Before this was in place, the record for the longest time without sleep was held by Randy Gardner. In 1964, aged 17, he stayed awake for 264 hours (11 days) and used absolutely no stimulants. Other claimants to the record include Maureen Weston, who in 1977 reportedly stayed awake for 449 hours during a rocking-chair competition, and Tony Wright, who live-streamed his sleepless feast of over 264 hours from a bar in Penzance, Cornwall, in 2007.

The largest sleepover recorded by Guinness World Records was on 27 September 2014, with 2,004 Girl Guides in their pyjamas during a camp in Cheshire, UK.

CERTIFICATE

for staying awake
the longest

is proudly presented to

Maureen Weston

---

*Who in 1977 reportedly stayed
awake for 449 hours during
a rocking-chair competition.*

DOES POOR SLEEP CONTRIBUTE
to Alzheimer's disease?

Several studies have found a link between insomnia and an increased risk of dementia. In his book *Why We Sleep*, neuroscientist Matthew Walker argues that sleep disorders often precede Alzheimer's and can be a warning sign of it developing.

Alzheimer's is the result of amyloid plaques building up in the brain. It could be that lack of sleep causes amyloids to accumulate. A University of Rochester study in 2019 found that deep NREM sleep helped to 'deep clean' the brain, removing toxic proteins like amyloid.

Walker and others suggest that a cruel cycle may take hold in which poor sleep causes amyloid plaques to build up, resulting in more sleep problems and yet more amyloid. Or, to put it more positively, improving your sleep may help deep clean your brain better and so lower your risk of Alzheimer's.

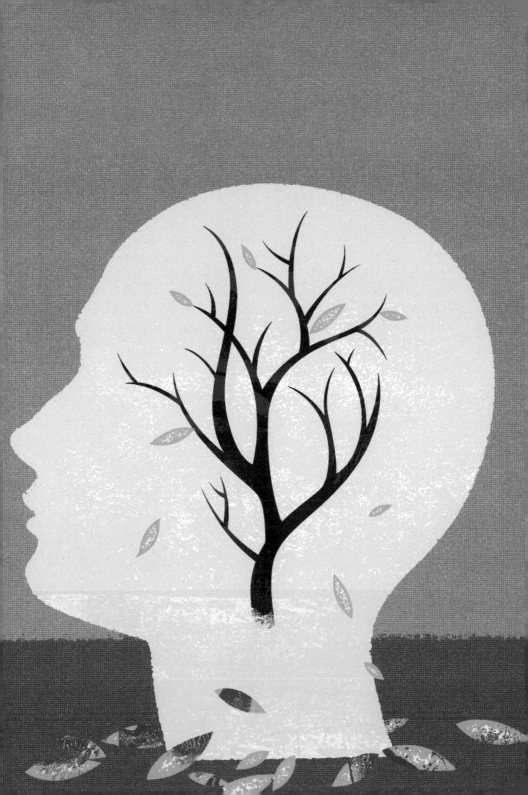

WHAT HAPPENS IF YOU DON'T SLEEP?

No wonder sleep deprivation is used as a means of torture – it debilitates almost every mental faculty of a person.

Sleep is such a fundamental state – it influences body-wide processes right down to the cellular level and refreshes the brain's capacity to face another day.

What results from a total lack of shut-eye is someone who is emotionally unstable, cannot accurately recall information and can hardly understand simple instructions, let alone undertake any logical reasoning. In extreme cases, hallucinations follow, often accompanied by suicidal thoughts.

A study showed that one night of sleep deprivation doubled the likelihood of someone confessing to something they'd not actually done.

Up all night – the second wind

Have you ever stayed up all night and then gone to work or college the next day? If so, you will have noticed that once you struggled past the new day's sunrise you didn't feel that bad in the morning, but the afternoon was a head-nodding period of blurred vision and brain fog.

The twin systems governing sleep – circadian rhythm and adenosine – help to explain this second wind on day two. While adenosine levels keep rising in your body, the body rhythms march ever onwards with their consequent morning peaks and afternoon troughs of alertness. Come late afternoon and evening, the combined sleep forces hit you head-on and slumber is immediate.

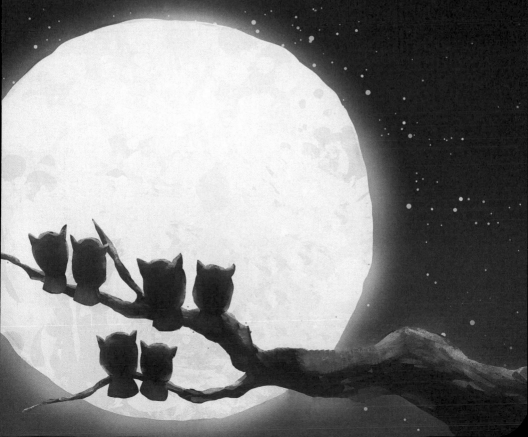

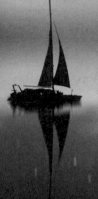

n World

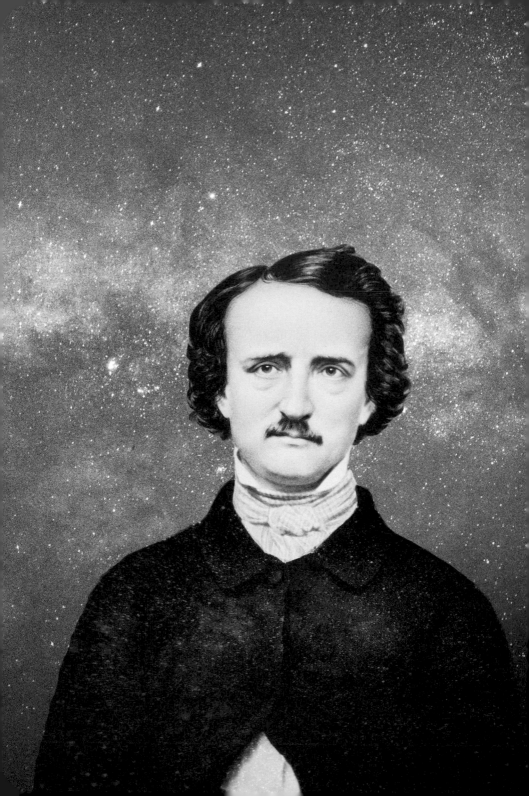

All That We See Or Seem Is But A Dream Within A Dream

Edgar Allan Poe, from the poem
'A Dream Within a Dream'

Dreaming is good for you

It's a curious thing. Why have we evolved to send ourselves into a state of unconsciousness for a long period every day? During your nightly cycles of sleep, you're totally and utterly vulnerable. There must be an advantage to gain. The nightly hallucinations of dreaming have a function, too, or so scientists think.

It's easy to rate the types of sleep – NREM and REM sleep – over one another. Surely the restorative slow-wave NREM sleep is more vital than the sleep where our eyes flicker beneath their lids? But all sleep is vital. And while the early cycles of sleep put NREM at their core, as we move through the night REM periods get progressively longer.

Recent research has shown that REM sleep – the time we have the most memorable and vivid dreams – is essential for learning, memory and creative thinking.

Healing via Dreams

The parts of the brain that deal with emotions are up to 30 per cent more active in REM sleep than during waking hours. Such a super-emotional brain, combined with powered-down sectors in logic and rational thought, serves to benefit our emotional and mental health.

In his book, *Why We Sleep*, Matthew Walker says:

'REM sleep dreaming offers a form of overnight therapy . . . takes the painful sting out of difficult, emotional episodes you have experienced during the day, offering emotional resolution when you awake the next morning.'

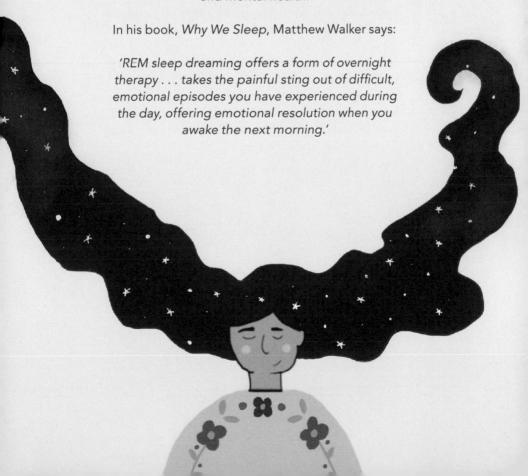

DREAM MORE,
Be Creative

REM sleep also allows the brain to meld memories together in new and novel ways – dreaming allows us to think outside the box, promoting problem solving and creative thinking. It's no surprise that many great and revolutionary ideas simply popped into the dreamer's brain during or after sleep.

In the few minutes on waking but before getting up, have you ever experienced a wondrous clarity of thought? Sparkling solutions surface effortlessly to issues that have been circling round and round in your brain. In those moments, you are reaping the benefits of dream sleep.

'It is a common experience that a problem difficult at night is resolved in the morning after the committee of sleep has worked on it.'

— John Steinbeck

World Sleep Day

When: Held every year on the Friday before the vernal equinox in spring (mid-March).

Who: The World Sleep Day Committee of the World Sleep Society founded the annual awareness event.

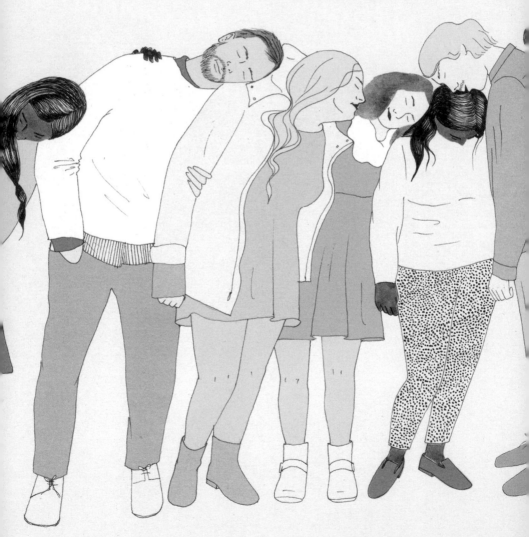

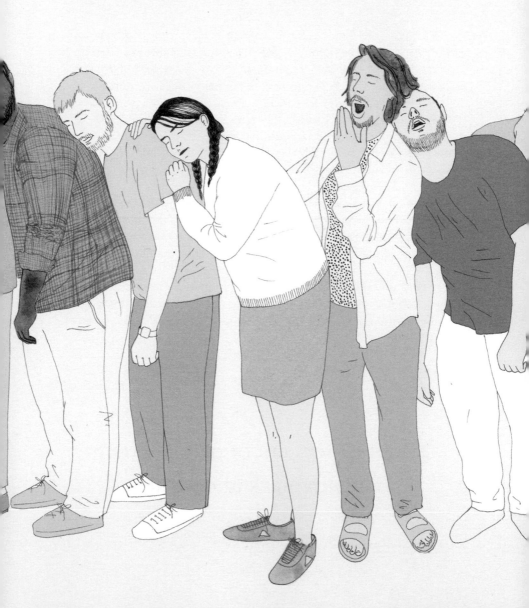

Why: To celebrate sleep as well as to champion sleep's importance and highlight sleep-related issues.

Follow #WorldSleepDay to discover how the world is celebrating all things sleep.

Black-and-white dreams
– so last century

Today, most people dream in colour. But it wasn't always so. Go back to the 1940s, and studies then revealed how 75 per cent of dreamers 'never' or 'rarely' experienced colourful nocturnal adventures.

A 2008 study found, too, that people born in the early 1950s who grew up before the widespread availability of colour TVs reported dreaming in black and white a quarter of the time. Whereas those aged 25 and under hardly ever dreamed in shades of grey.

How we consume visual imagery as children – in black and white or full-on colour – appears to translate into the tints of our dreams. So, with a typical LED TV or smartphone displaying millions of colours, could we be seeing the end of monochromatic dreamscapes?

It may simply be that some of us don't remember the colours of a dream. But one theory links colourful dreams with creativity – the more creative you are, the more colourful sleepy adventures you have.

About 12 per cent of people dream only in black and white.

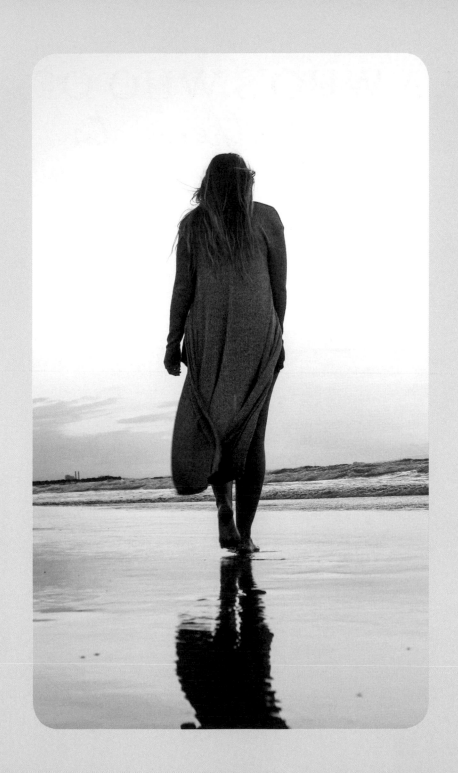

A WHO'S WHO OF
Dream theorists

Since ancient times, people have wanted to know more about the mysterious dream state. Below is a flavour of the varied modern ideas proposed to explain why we dream.

Sigmund Freud (1856–1939)
The founder of psychoanalysis had a theory of dreams as a form of wish fulfilment – repressed desires could be acted out in the sphere of dreams without fear of being unacceptable. Perhaps because he lived in the days of sexual repression, Freud's ideas focused mainly on desire.

Carl Jung (1875–1961)
A former student of Freud, Jung broke with Freud's ideas and followed a different path. He believed that dreams reveal more than they conceal. In Jung's mind, dreams were a natural expression of imagination, seen through a series of symbols and metaphors. He suggested, too, that dreams integrate the conscious and unconscious minds.

Antti Revonsuo (1963–)
A Finnish psychologist and neuroscientist best known for his 'threat simulation theory' of dreams. Stemming from the similarities between the way the brain fires up during REM sleep and in the 'fight or flight' response, he believes that dreams are a rehearsal for evading threats in real life. The work you do in your dreams keeps you safe during waking hours.

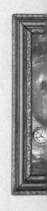

'What would an ocean be without a monster lurking in the dark? It would be like sleep without dreams.'

– Werner Herzog

J. Allan Hobson (1933–) and Robert McCarley (1937–2017)
In the 1970s, these two psychiatrists proposed what's known as 'the activation–synthesis hypothesis' – a revolutionary idea at the time suggesting that dreams are simply the brain trying to make sense of random electrical activity. This theory proposed that dreams don't have meaning, but the waking brain tries to create stories without being aware of doing it.

'I have noticed that dreams are as simple or as complicated as the dreamer is himself, only they are always a little bit ahead of the dreamer's consciousness.'

– Carl Jung

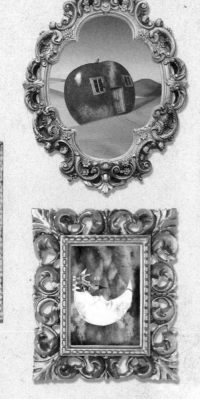

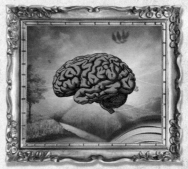

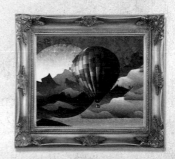

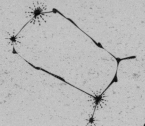
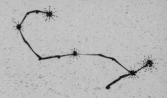

Dream journalling

Dreams can expand the way we see the world, help us solve problems and bring clarity. Get to know yourself better and connect with your subconscious thoughts and feelings by chronicling details about your dreams.

1. Write on waking – Keep a journal and a pen by your bed and capture your dreams immediately on waking. Don't worry if your hastily scribbled notes need to be transcribed later, it's vital to get the details as soon after waking as possible.

2. Be patient – Don't worry if you can barely recollect any details of your dreams. Write down what you remember, even if it seems a strange detail – maybe just a feeling or a colour. Open up to what's being revealed.

3. Record every day – Turn this practice into a habit. This can help you remember your dreams more easily and, what's more, they'll offer fresh insight and new perspective.

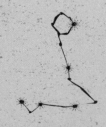

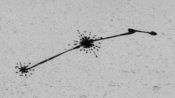
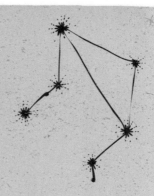

4. Be specific – Write the details down even if they seem unimportant. A seemingly trivial detail can sometimes open the door to more memories.

5. Allow weirdness – Dreams are naturally bizarre. Resist filling in the gaps, creating a plot or forcing it to all make sense. Just write what you remember.

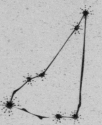

6. Use your own style – Write in whatever form you like – be that bullet points, narrative prose, a stream of consciousness or as pictures. Enjoy the process. Give yourself 5 to 10 minutes and do what you can in that amount of time.

7. Assign a title – Take a moment to sum up your dream and give it a title. This step offers closure on last night's dream before you move on with your day.

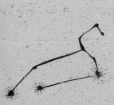
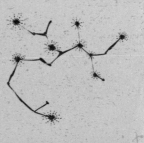

Your Dream Record

Date _____

Who were you in your dream?

Who else was in your dream?

Where were you? What did it look like?
What were you doing?

How were you interacting with your environment and others?

What symbols, objects, animals, colours, shapes and textures did you notice?

What were you thinking? What were you feeling?

Close your eyes. Take a deep breath and come up with a title for your dream (please only do this after you've recorded all the above details):

The bizarre world of dreams

Many dreams are strange, even downright weird. Bizarre nocturnal imaginings of scenes in which you become a superhero of sorts – you can fly, breathe underwater, leap between skyscrapers, or slow down the fabric of time – seem totally normal while your eyes are closed.

But what makes these fleeting night-time episodes so unreal? The brain's pattern of activity transforms during the dark hours – certain parts are more active while others quieten or shut off completely.

During dreaming, we can no longer access memories of life events, though we can still grab general memories about people and places. The brain becomes super-emotional and, at the same time, the rational brain that controls decision-making powers down. As such, our imagination is allowed to run riot with little input from logic or reasoning thoughts – unrealness can abound.

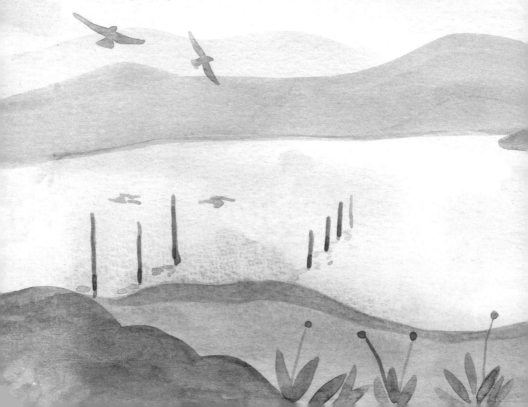

Nightmarish scenarios

Some people are more prone to nightmares than others, research shows. One theory suggests that those who often suffer from nightmares turn out to have greater empathy when awake. And this heightened sensitivity gives them a creative edge, both in their dreaming and in their waking lives. Imagery rehearsal training – where a person rewrites their nightmare, giving it a happier ending and visualizing this every time before they sleep – maximizes the vivid imaginations of such people.

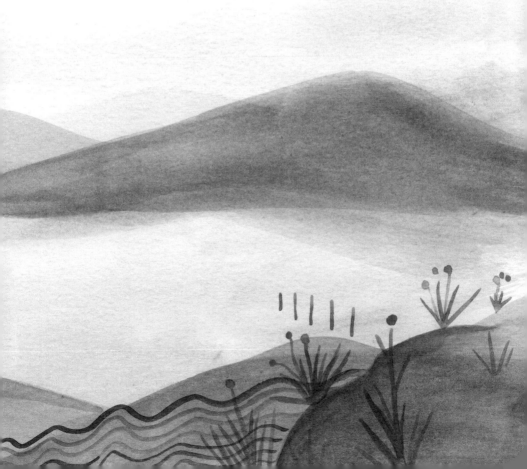

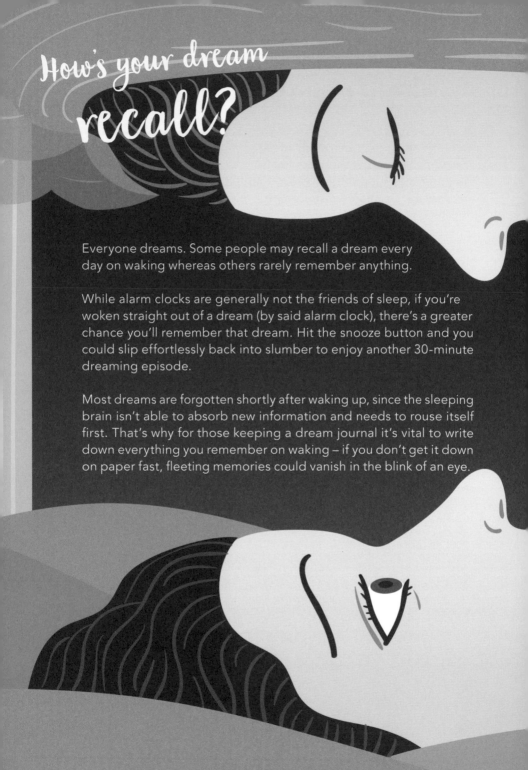

How's your dream recall?

Everyone dreams. Some people may recall a dream every day on waking whereas others rarely remember anything.

While alarm clocks are generally not the friends of sleep, if you're woken straight out of a dream (by said alarm clock), there's a greater chance you'll remember that dream. Hit the snooze button and you could slip effortlessly back into slumber to enjoy another 30-minute dreaming episode.

Most dreams are forgotten shortly after waking up, since the sleeping brain isn't able to absorb new information and needs to rouse itself first. That's why for those keeping a dream journal it's vital to write down everything you remember on waking – if you don't get it down on paper fast, fleeting memories could vanish in the blink of an eye.

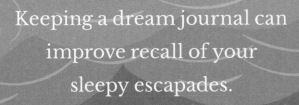

Keeping a dream journal can improve recall of your sleepy escapades.

You'd expect perhaps that the more bizarre the dream, the easier it is to recall, but research shows that it's those night-time adventures with strongly emotional content and organized plot lines that are more easily remembered.

In 2014, scientists discovered that a particular part of the brain – known as the temporoparietal junction (or TPJ for short) – is more active in 'high dream recallers' compared with 'low dream recallers'; the TPJ is the part of the brain that reacts to noise and other external stimuli. The 'high dream recallers' also woke up twice as often during the night.

The combination of being awake for brief spells and an active TPJ helps the 'high dream recallers' encode dreams into memory – they can recall more easily what they were just dreaming about.

Sleep scientists can now predict much about people's dreams before the dreamers reveal the facts themselves.

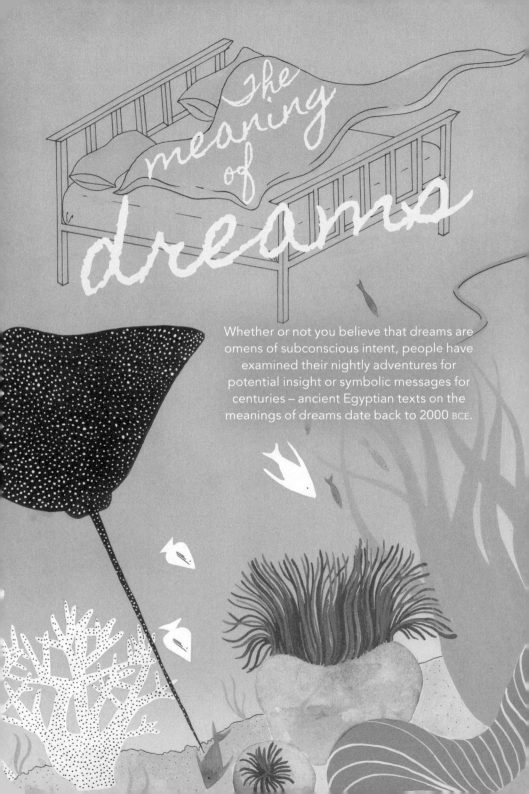

the meaning of dreams

Whether or not you believe that dreams are omens of subconscious intent, people have examined their nightly adventures for potential insight or symbolic messages for centuries – ancient Egyptian texts on the meanings of dreams date back to 2000 BCE.

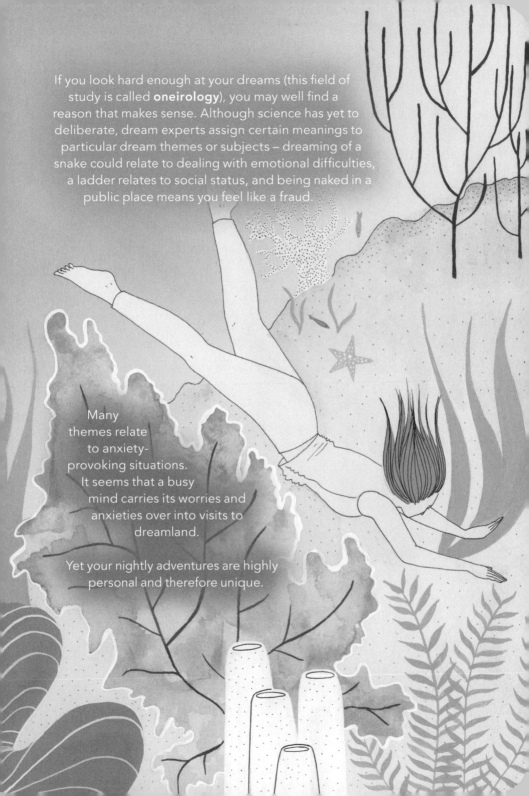

If you look hard enough at your dreams (this field of study is called **oneirology**), you may well find a reason that makes sense. Although science has yet to deliberate, dream experts assign certain meanings to particular dream themes or subjects – dreaming of a snake could relate to dealing with emotional difficulties, a ladder relates to social status, and being naked in a public place means you feel like a fraud.

Many themes relate to anxiety-provoking situations. It seems that a busy mind carries its worries and anxieties over into visits to dreamland.

Yet your nightly adventures are highly personal and therefore unique.

TOP 10 | MOST COMMON RECURRING *Dreams*

A US survey in 2016 came up with the following common dream themes. How many resonate with you?

If a recurring dream changes over time, or disappears altogether, that's most likely a sign that the problem's been resolved.

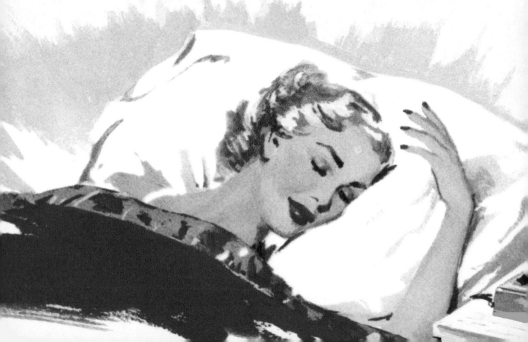

1. FALLING

2. BEING CHASED

3. BEING BACK IN SCHOOL

4. BEING UNPREPARED FOR
   A TEST OR IMPORTANT EVENT

5. FLYING

6. HAVING SEX WITH SOMEONE
   YOU SHOULDN'T HAVE

7. ENCOUNTERING A PERSON
   WHO HAS DIED IN REAL LIFE

8. DEATH

9. HAVING YOUR TEETH FALL OUT

10. BEING LOST

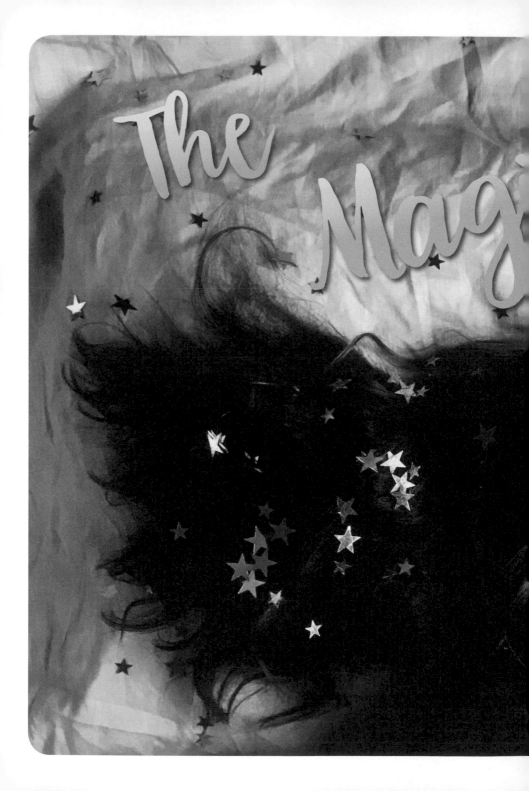

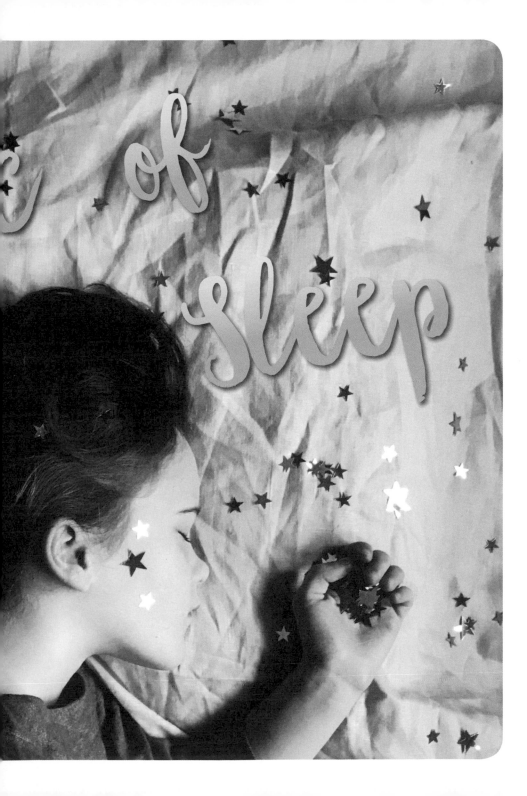

Learning in your sleep – is it possible?

Simply slotting that holiday phrase book under your pillow isn't going to give you the lingo to decipher a Greek menu or negotiate a Spanish car park. But scientific studies show that while you sleep your brain is reinforcing memories and forming new ones.

Learn new associations
Scientists in Israel arranged for a group of smokers to stay overnight in a sleep lab, where the team exposed their volunteers to the smell of cigarettes plus an awful odour of rotten fish or rotten eggs. Less than a week after the experiment, the participants were smoking 30 per cent less. To confirm it was sleep that was special in creating the new associations, the study was also done while people were awake, but that had no effect on smoking rates.

Sleep is crucial for learning and memory formation. NREM sleep in particular is vital for consolidating memories.

Swot up on foreign vocab

Subliminal swotting was demonstrated by German researchers who were teaching Dutch to German natives. As part of the study, while the subjects were asleep, the research team played recorded Dutch words to one group; the other was left to sleep in silence. When they were tested, the group exposed to the sounds of words during the night were better able to identify the new Dutch vocab.

Improve musical skills

Researchers in another study taught people to play a simple melody on the guitar. All volunteers got to nap afterwards. One group was exposed to the same melody while they slept and the other group simply snoozed away. Despite being unaware of having heard the music during their sleep, the participants who were exposed to the music went on to play the guitar melody much better than the other group.

So be sure to snooze after learning anything new and let sleep do its magical work.

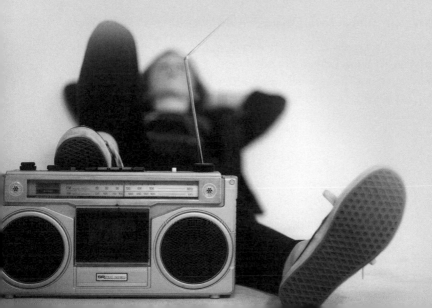

IS SLEEPSTORMING THE NEW BRAINSTORMING?

Tap into the power of your brain while you're asleep; while you snooze, your brain is active but working in a completely different way from when you're awake. Boost your odds of generating ideas during slumber by 'sleepstorming' – like brainstorming but done solo and while you're asleep. Try these simple hacks.

Keep a notebook handy – and write down your dreams.

Get into the habit of writing down your dreams – and any ideas they might trigger – immediately on waking and almost before you are fully awake.

Ask your subconscious the question you're trying to answer.

'Never go to sleep without a request to your subconscious,' advised Thomas Edison, the great inventor. So, brief or prime your subconscious. Before falling asleep, pose yourself the *question du jour* before switching off and focusing on something else, such as reading or a relaxation technique.

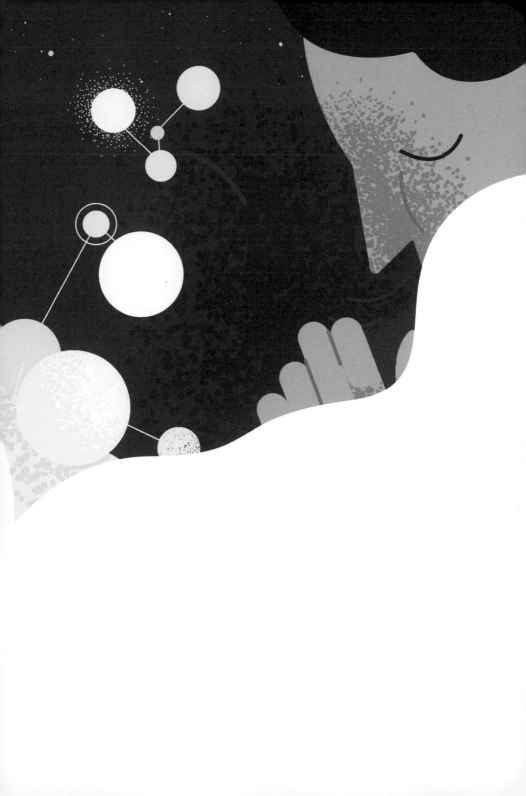

The world of lucid dreaming

Very few people successfully manage to do this, but if you want to try it, the first step to lucid dreaming is to pay more attention to your dreams.

While some people want to dive in and control their dreams, that's not all of what lucid dreaming is about. Instead, lucid dreamers learn to become more self-aware, all the while exploring new possibilities within a dreamscape.

Lucid dreaming for beginners

1. Go to bed and set a gentle alarm for 5 hours later; you need some restorative deep sleep first.
2. On waking with your alarm, resist the urge to roll over and don't move.
3. Simply lie there and relax. You need to be conscious but allow your body to enter a sleep paralysis. This stage can feel a bit scary, as many people report feeling like they have a weight pressing on their chest. Don't panic.
4. Within a minute or so, you should be able to experience a lucid dream.
5. The next morning when you wake up, record as many details as you can.

Greek philosopher Aristotle's treatise *On Dreams* could be the first record of lucid dreaming; in it he describes his self-awareness during a dream.

Your Dream Record

Date_____

Who were you in your dream? Who else was in your dream?

Where were you? What did it look like? What were you doing?

How were you interacting with your environment and others?

What symbols, objects, animals, colours, shapes and textures
did you notice?

What were you thinking? What were you feeling?

Close your eyes. Take a deep breath and come up with a title for your
dream (please only do this after you've recorded all the above details):

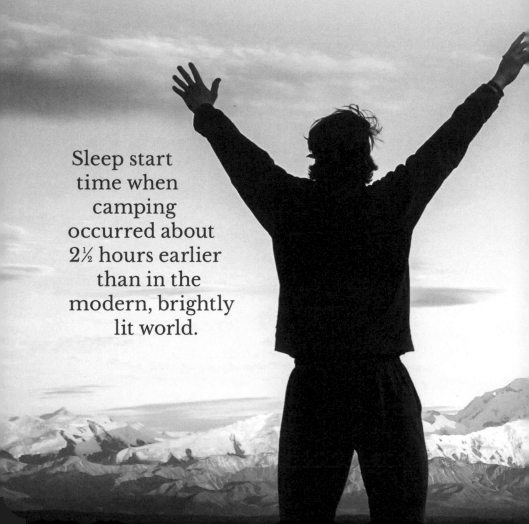

Pitch black: camping to

Since we know that modern life has disengaged us from the long-evolved relationship with the light and dark of the day, it's great to discover that there's a simple (and non-expensive) fix – a 'back to nature' camping holiday.

Sleep start time when camping occurred about 2½ hours earlier than in the modern, brightly lit world.

reset your circadian clock

A team of researchers at the University of Colorado designed a study to confirm how life delays circadian rhythm and the onset of sleep in those living in modern environments, with bright electric lighting, LED-lit devices and modern working hours. They wanted to see, too, if people could adjust their circadian clocks with the seasons.

They arranged for participants to go camping in the Rocky Mountains for a 2-week session in winter and a weekend stint in summer – no devices or torches were allowed, only sunlight, moonlight and firelight. What they discovered was that they quickly adjusted to shorter days and longer nights in winter and to longer days and shorter nights in summer.

Sleeping in a tent – with its translucent nylon shell – allows sunlight in, so you'll be up with the sun and in bed come sundown. So, if you feel that your busy life has taken over, grab a sleeping bag and tent and head for the hills. Resetting your biological rhythm generator will have you coming home feeling refreshed and with a better sleeping schedule built in for weeks to come.

Could camping be a way to future-proof sleep and reconnect with the daily and annual cycles of nature?

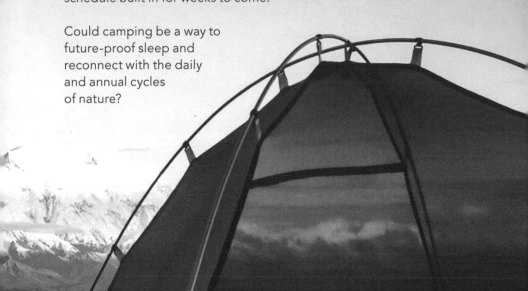

Sleep for a competitive edge

Tennis ace Roger Federer apparently sleeps for up to 12 hours a day, Usain Bolt grabs at least 10 hours shut-eye each night and many basketball players nap before games.

When it comes to being at the top of your game, sleep is just as important as nutrition and training schedules for athletes and professional sportspeople. So much so that, since 2005, sleep coaches are often integral members of the entourage, helping cyclists, runners and footballers, among others, to achieve the very best of what's possible.

AT LONDON'S 2012 OLYMPIC GAMES, THE BRITISH CYCLING TEAM SMASHED WORLD RECORDS. EACH MEMBER OF THE TEAM HAD THEIR OWN SLEEP KIT.

Performing at the elite level of any sport requires a body in supreme physical condition and a super-sharp brain. A lack of sleep causes not only reductions in stamina and strength but also slower reaction times and reflexes and less focus. Getting enough sleep will give a sprinter, for example, the best advantage out of the starting blocks.

Hours of intense physical exercise put great demand on muscles and soft tissues. Given that the body repairs itself while we sleep, it's perhaps no surprise that elite sportspeople strategically nap to aid recovery after heavy training as well as to revitalize ahead of competitions.

When milliseconds can decide the difference between a medal and fourth place, every athlete is looking for any competitive edge. For many, this edge is sleep.

Basketball players who bagged an extra 2 hours of shut-eye could sprint faster, react faster and their throws were significantly more accurate.

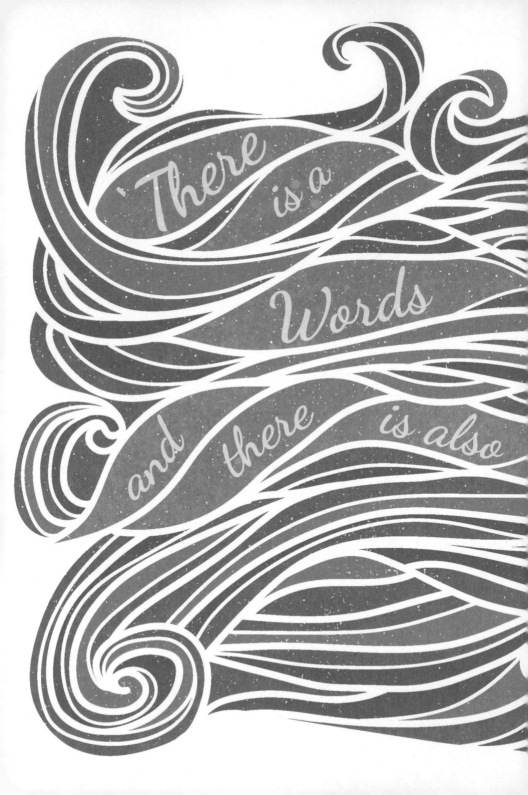

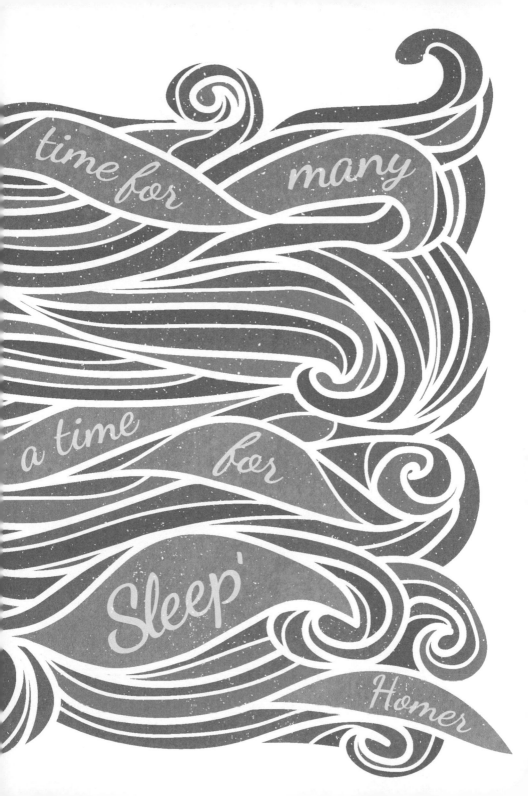

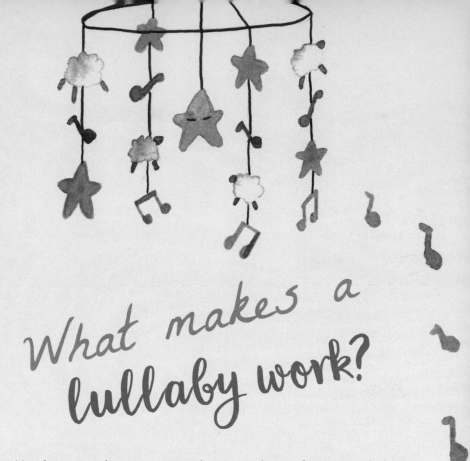

What makes a lullaby work?

Nearly every culture appears to have a tradition of singing to babies and young children, usually accompanied by a rocking motion, to get them to the land of nod. Children – and adults, too – find it hard to resist the drowsiness and heavy eyelids that soon appear on hearing a lullaby.

In some societies the words of the song itself are a means of passing on oral traditions. Lullabies help boost the bond between parent and child, as babies have a strong preference for their mother's voice over others. The words of lullabies can sometimes be mournful, as in the Gaelic 'Ba Ba Mo Leanabh Beag', about the Irish potato famine, so they might also have a cathartic role in voicing the fears of parents.

Most lullabies are written in triple metre or 6/8 time, which produces a swinging motion. Such rocking imitates the movement of the baby in the womb and, along with the repetitive nature of the songs, has a soothing effect.

Simplicity is best, and lullabies are usually confined to about five notes and sung in a high-pitched voice. It seems that babies prefer the harmonies of consonant intervals rather than dissonant intervals. A tempo of 60 beats per minute is best – similar to the beating of a human heart – reminding the baby of the lubb-dupp background rhythm of their mother's womb.

Research suggests that infants prefer lullabies that are sung unaccompanied by musical instruments.

Lullabies are soothing for adults as well as children and are an effective way of countering stress.

Sleep Music

Calm has used the soothing tones of Stephen Fry to read lullabies for adults. Other drowsiness-inducing soundscapes on Calm feature the sounds of ocean waves, heavy rain, a campfire burning, a babbling brook, a waterfall, white noise, sounds of a train ride, sounds of city streets, thunderstorms, pink noise, a purring cat, whale song, the chirruping of evening crickets, an oscillating fan, a heartbeat and even a washing machine.

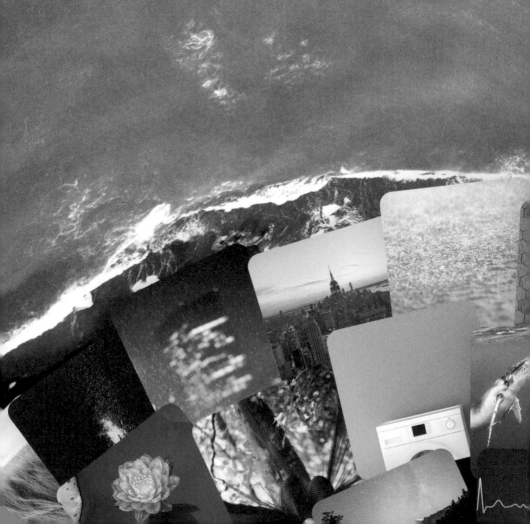

Head over to the following link to listen to an excerpt from Calm as you drift into dreamland.

www.calm.com/sleep

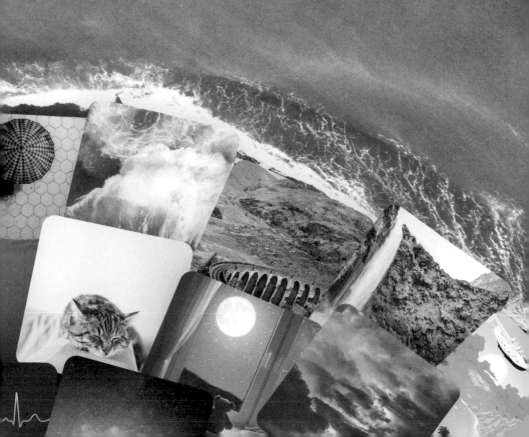

How Meditation and

In the quest for healthy sleep, meditation can be an extremely helpful practice. Let's explore why.

It's common for many of us to rush through our day and then climb into bed only to discover that our active mind keeps us awake for hours. We'll lie in bed ruminating over an argument, worrying about world events, or fixating on a project that's due tomorrow. Whatever challenges we're facing, they are sure to rise to the surface come bedtime.

That's why meditating before bed can be so helpful. Meditation can help quiet our overactive mind and set the stage for peaceful sleep. When we stop and concentrate our attention on the breath, rather than our anxious thoughts, both our body and mind begin to settle. Body scan practices in particular are very helpful because they direct our attention from thought to sensation.

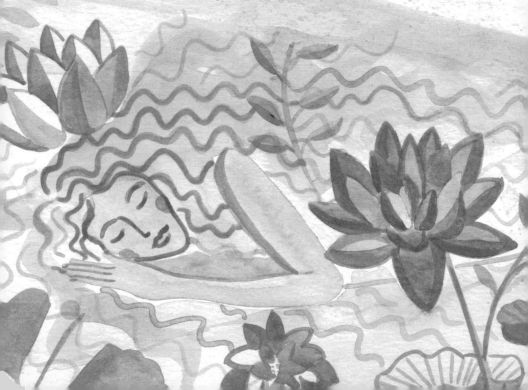

Mindfulness help sleep

Meditation also helps us cultivate the skill of non-reactivity. It's common to struggle to fall asleep, and then find ourselves anxious precisely because of our sleeplessness. We lie awake worrying about how poor sleep will impact our energy levels or productivity the next day. Then the stress of not being able to sleep ends up keeping us awake. Non-reactivity, one of the primary teachings in meditation, means that we learn how to *be* with our experience without reacting to it. When lying awake, we simply note that we're awake, without adding further anxious thoughts. By letting go of the pressure to fall asleep, we're able to relax, and *that's* when sleep naturally happens.

So on those nights when sleep doesn't come easily, call on your meditation practice to quieten your busy thoughts and relax your body, leading the way to deep, restful sleep.

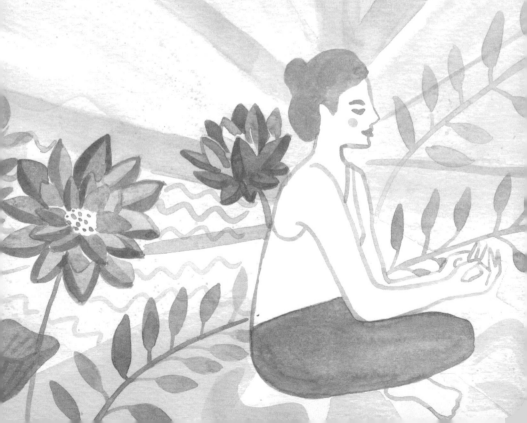

A sleep meditation

*There are different ways to enjoy this practice.
You can review these instructions, commit them to memory and
then walk through them yourself before bed. You can have someone
read this script to you. Or even feel free to record yourself reading
this practice and listen to it at bedtime.*

Welcome to this relaxing meditation to
help you drift off to dreamland.

To start, find a comfortable position on your bed,
lying down on your back.

Let your shoulders drop naturally, and allow your
hands to rest by your sides in an easy, effortless way.
If you'd prefer, you can place both hands on your
belly. Choose whatever position feels
most comfortable.

Let your feet fall apart naturally, and close your eyes.

Gently, bring your attention to your body,
sweeping your awareness from your head to your feet,
tuning into all sensations. Notice if there are any parts
that feel tight, and if there are, take a few deep
breaths, and on each exhale, see if you can invite
those areas to relax.

Now allow the breath to fall into a natural rhythm, and for these next few exhales, let go of thoughts, let go of worries, let go of anything that pulls on your attention. Do your best to be right here, right now.

Focus your attention on the sensation of your belly rising and falling, rising and falling.

Feel the breath flowing in and flowing out . . .

And now, begin a body scan practice, scanning each part of your body, starting from the top of your head, all the way to the tip of your toes. Slowly, shift your attention throughout the length of your body, relaxing and releasing each part.

On each inhale and each exhale, relax and release, over and over.

With each breath you take, feel the weight of your body sinking into your bed.

Allow a feeling of peace and relaxation to flow through your body as you fall into a deep, restful sleep.

by Tamara Levitt
(Head of Mindfulness at Calm)

How *grat* helps yo

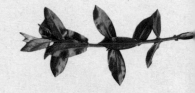

Committing ideas or thoughts to paper has a remarkable effect – it makes them real. And research has shown that writing a gratitude journal for just 15 minutes a day can help you sleep better and for longer.

If you're a worrier or suffer with anxiety, you'll know all too well how thoughts of tomorrow's potential problems or what you failed to get done today can ruminate and delay your trip to dreamland. You need to embrace the idea of gratitude.

Being grateful is an aspect of mindfulness where you live more in the present, notice the good things in life and are thankful for those. Cultivating an attitude of gratitude throughout the day is known to boost happiness and life satisfaction, as well as filling your mind with positive thoughts as you drift off to sleep.

And don't be shy. Express this gratitude – show that colleague that you really appreciated her help, thank the fitness trainer for a fantastic class or a friend for a thoughtful text.

Every time you look for the positive and are thankful, you reinforce what's positive about your life. Being mindful of such things calms your mind at bedtime, so you'll nod off faster, slumber longer and wake refreshed.

Get the gratitude habit

- Complete a gratitude journal ideally throughout the day or at the end of each day – try to include three to five things for which you're thankful every day. Either choose a small handy-sized book to carry with you, or download an app for easier jotting down across the day.

- Verbalize and express your thanks out loud at least once a week – whether it's a 'thank you' for your morning latte or for some kindness from a stranger.

- Thank those who have made a difference to your life throughout the year. No expensive gifts or gestures are needed – a handwritten card or letter speaks volumes about your heartfelt thanks.

Three things happy

Every night before you go to sleep, name three things that happened that day that made you feel happy, then think of three things that made you feel good about yourself. Write them down or say them aloud, it's up to you. It's a great way to reinforce a healthy self-image and a positive mindset and ensure you go to sleep with happy thoughts in your head. This works brilliantly with children, too, and has the added benefit that you get to hear a bit about their day and the things that genuinely bring them joy – often surprising things. Share your own list with them, so that they can hear about your day as well.

that made you

1

2

3

It's storytelling

– but not as you know it

The first bedtime story generated by artificial intelligence (AI) is also the first new Brothers Grimm fairy tale in 200 years.

The story – *The Princess and the Fox* – is the product of a predictive text algorithm that was fed the stories of Jacob and Wilhelm Grimm and trained to mimic their style. It's now part of the Sleep Story collection on Calm.

The new story is a collaborative effort between computers and humans. A group of writers, artists and programmers that go under the moniker Botnik use machine intelligence to create new forms of writing.

So, from the long-dead German brothers who gave us our standard versions of such age-old oral tales as *Cinderella*, *Rapunzel*, *Hansel and Gretel*, *Little Red Riding Hood*, *Snow White* and *Sleeping Beauty* now comes *The Lost Grimm Fairy Tale*.

The story itself tells of a king, a magical golden horse, a forlorn princess and a poor miller's son. A talking fox helps the lowly miller's son to rescue the beautiful princess from the fate of having to marry a dreadful prince who she does not love.

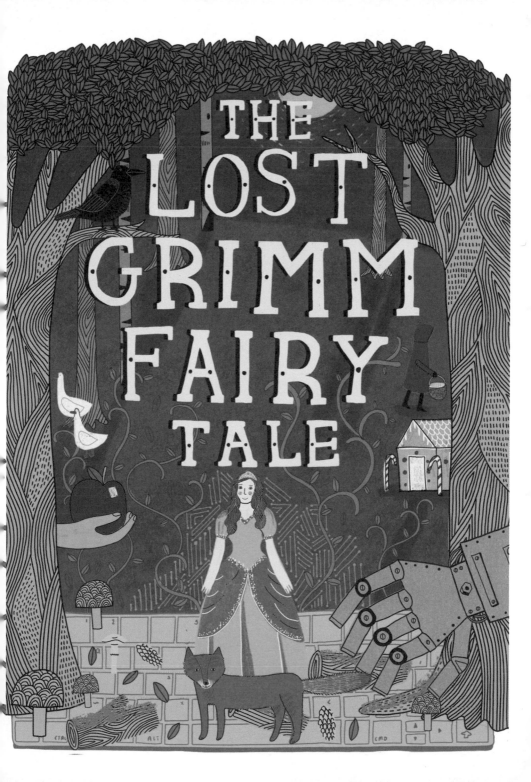

THE FUTURE
of SLEEP

Since sleep became the new buzzword of health, all sorts of gadgets promising you the ultimate good night's sleep have appeared – from the actual bed and pillow to sleep-tracking devices and lights that mimic the sun.

Snore preventers

Imagine being buzzed by a band across your chest every time you shifted into a back-lying sleeping position. Doesn't sound like the formula for a well-rested night, does it? But for people suffering from obstructive sleep apnoea, such devices can stop them snoring and halt the characteristic pause in breathing. As a result, sufferers should wake feeling refreshed rather than tired all the time. Another wireless tracker is a stamp-sized sticker that you pop on your forehead; it measures oxygen levels in your blood and tries to spot when you stop breathing.

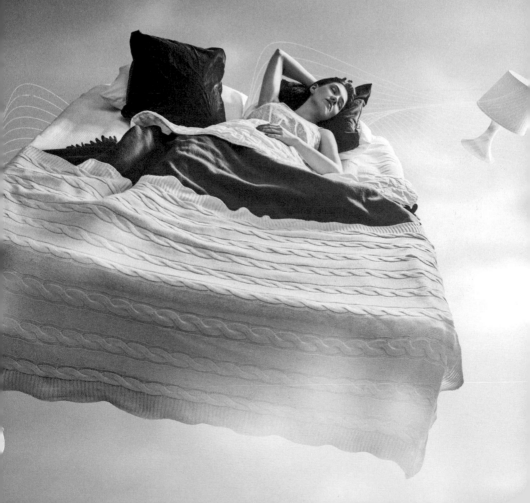

Orthosomnia –
the anxiety created through becoming
obsessed about getting the perfect
night's sleep.

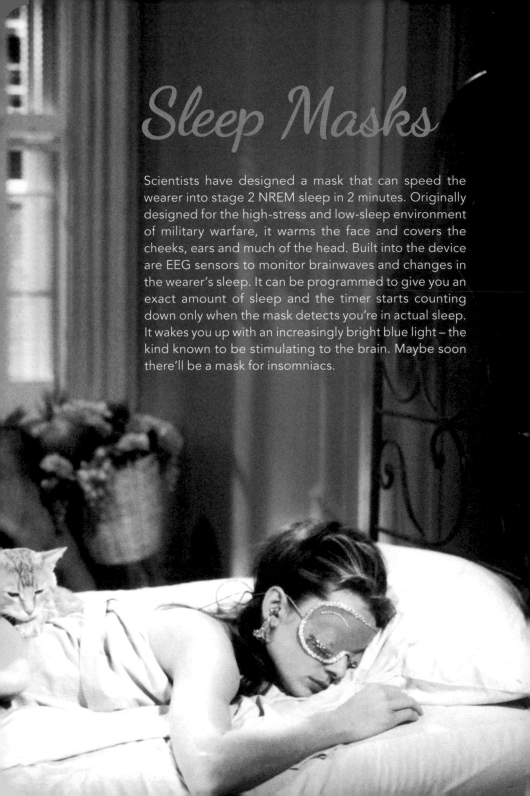

Sleep Masks

Scientists have designed a mask that can speed the wearer into stage 2 NREM sleep in 2 minutes. Originally designed for the high-stress and low-sleep environment of military warfare, it warms the face and covers the cheeks, ears and much of the head. Built into the device are EEG sensors to monitor brainwaves and changes in the wearer's sleep. It can be programmed to give you an exact amount of sleep and the timer starts counting down only when the mask detects you're in actual sleep. It wakes you up with an increasingly bright blue light – the kind known to be stimulating to the brain. Maybe soon there'll be a mask for insomniacs.

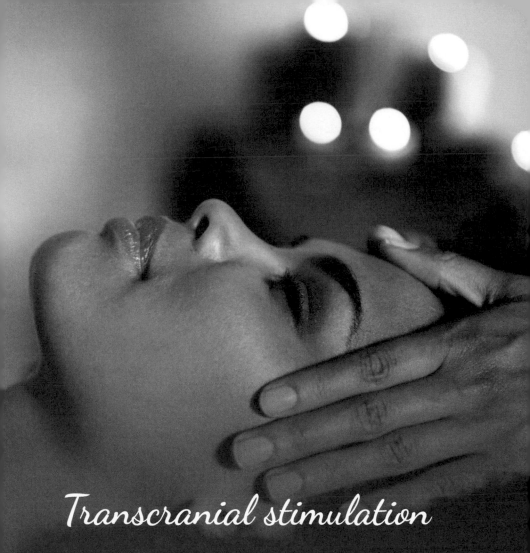

Transcranial stimulation

It may be the stuff of science fiction but manipulating brainwaves is already possible. Today, transcranial stimulators are being used as ways of nudging a person into good sleep patterns or into a certain level of sleep. One uses a weak electrical current (transcranial direct current stimulation), while another uses the power of magnets (transcranial magnetic stimulation). Researchers have been able to shift someone's sleep up into lighter sleep and down into deeper sleep, but since some of the machines required to do this are massive it'll be a while before you see such technology in the bedroom.

Suspended animation

Science fiction or science fact?
Sci-fi fans are familiar with transporting people through space in a sort of inanimate sleep during intergalactic or even interplanetary trips. But how close are we to being able to do this today?

Bears and their wintertime torpor have inspired SpaceWorks to design a craft for NASA to get humans all the way to Mars. If we could engineer humans to follow the same physiological conditions as the bear, we could slip into an unconscious state and wake up on Mars some six months later.

Could humans hack it, though? Many mammals hibernate, so there may well be scope for us to do the same. Doctors already exploit the use of cold temperatures when performing open heart surgery.

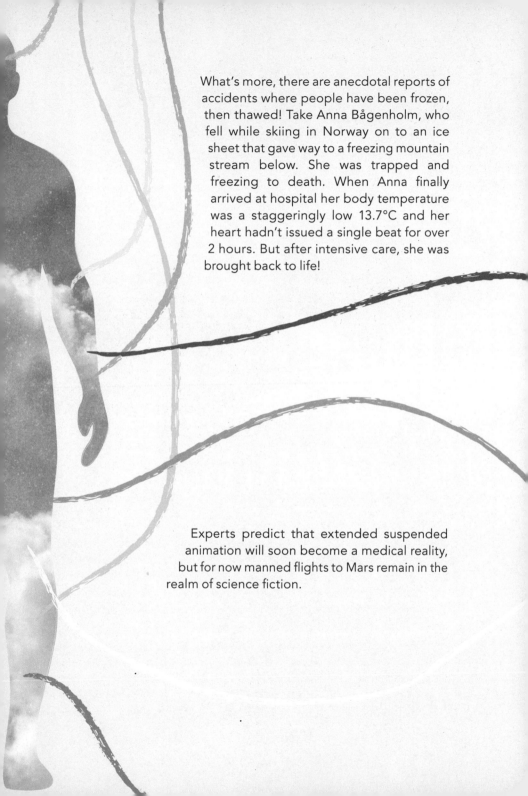

What's more, there are anecdotal reports of accidents where people have been frozen, then thawed! Take Anna Bågenholm, who fell while skiing in Norway on to an ice sheet that gave way to a freezing mountain stream below. She was trapped and freezing to death. When Anna finally arrived at hospital her body temperature was a staggeringly low 13.7°C and her heart hadn't issued a single beat for over 2 hours. But after intensive care, she was brought back to life!

Experts predict that extended suspended animation will soon become a medical reality, but for now manned flights to Mars remain in the realm of science fiction.

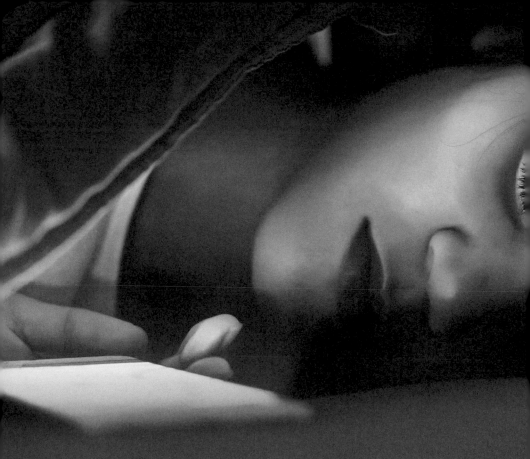

The rise and rise of Sleep Stories

Drifting off with the radio in the background is so old-school (though still a successful soporific). These days millions of people are regularly listening to podcasts, audiobooks and apps for their nightly dose of bedtime stories. Using your smartphone to unwind from a busy day and prepare yourself for slumber has never been so easy – a smart way to use this technology with sleep in mind.

To date, there have been a total of 150 million listens.

While Sleep Stories ranging from tales of travel to modern-day fairy tales to classics in shorter form are hugely popular, soundscapes – rain on city streets, waterfalls or train rides – are also widely used short cuts to shut-eye.

1 Search for Calm in your chosen app store

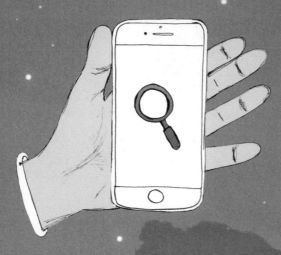

2 Download Calm

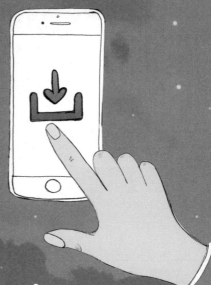

3 Open the app

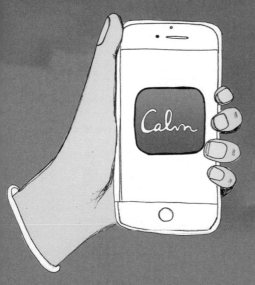

4 Enjoy

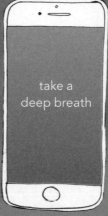

10 OF THE MOST POPULAR
Sleep Stories on Calm

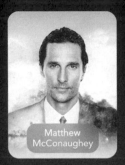

1. WONDER

(Narrated by Matthew McConaughey)

Join Matthew McConaughey for a dreamy story about the mysteries of the universe, in a heartfelt tale full of magic and wonder.

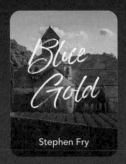

Stephen Fry

3. SERENITY OF THE SEA

(Narrated by Freema Agyeman)

Join actress Freema Agyeman for another enchanting journey through the magical kingdom of Lionwood.

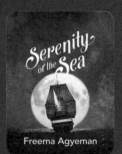

Freema Agyeman

2. BLUE GOLD

(Narrated by Stephen Fry)

Let master storyteller Stephen Fry take you on a serene journey through the lavender fields and sleepy villages of Provence.

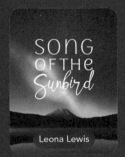

Leona Lewis

4. SONG OF THE SUNBIRD

(Narrated by Leona Lewis)

Follow the calming voice of Leona Lewis on this moonlit quest through the jungles of Kilimanjaro.

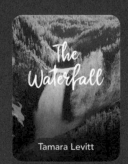

Tamara Levitt

5. THE WATERFALL

(Narrated by Tamara Levitt)

A soothing journey through nature to discover the source of a magnificent sound, narrated by Calm's own Tamara Levitt.

6. THE VELVETEEN RABBIT

(Narrated by Anna Acton)

The classic tale of a really splendid rabbit, read by British actress Anna Acton.

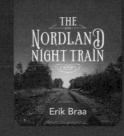

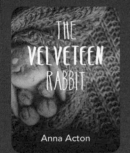

7. THE NORDLAND NIGHT TRAIN

(Narrated by Erik Braa)

Tonight, travel up the scenic coast of Norway aboard one of Europe's most breathtaking and remote railways.

8. CLOSE YOUR EYES SLEEPYPAWS

(Narrated by Philippa Alexander)

Join SleepyPaws in this dreamy tale set in the melodic world of Moshi Twilight Sleep Stories. (Produced by Calm in partnership with Moshi Twilight Sleep Stories, the Sleep Stories app for kids.)

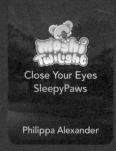

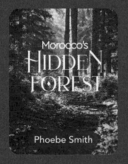

9. MOROCCO'S HIDDEN FOREST

(Narrated by Phoebe Smith)

Join author Phoebe Smith, Calm's Sleep Storyteller-in-Residence, for an enchanting journey to the sleepy hidden forests of Morocco.

10. THE NUTCRACKER

(Narrated by Larry Davis)

Tonight, travel to a world of magic and enchantment, as you drift off to this classic and beloved tale.

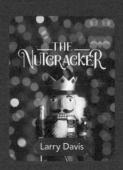

The art of writing people to sleep

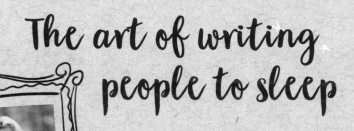

Here Phoebe Smith, Sleep Storyteller-in-Residence at Calm, tells her story of how she became 'the J. K. Rowling of "slow literature"'.

When I was a little girl, I remember seeing a book in my mum's study called *Words Were Originally Magic*. As a lover of the written word, and at that age also fascinated by all things supernatural, that phrase both captivated and puzzled me. How, I wondered, could the simple act of stringing together letters, words and phrases hold the same power as wizards and witches chanting spells and flicking wands?

Despite many people telling me it was impossible, I found my answer by becoming a writer and soon learned to wield my pen (or these days, my keyboard) with the same power as an enchantress.

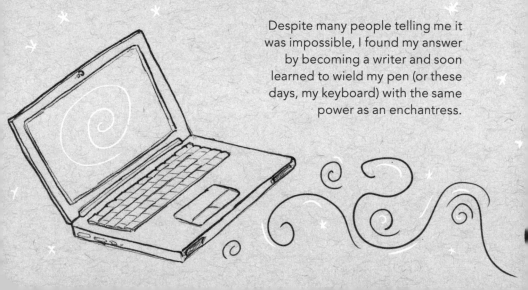

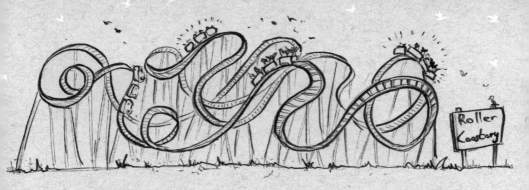

My specialist subjects are travel, nature and wildlife. Working for newspapers, magazines and radio stations around the world, I pen tales of my adventures designed to capture the imagination, to hurl readers onwards as though on a metaphorical roller coaster, gripping them with anticipation right until I hit the brakes at the end.

Until a couple of years ago, I would always make it my mission when writing to ensure that, once a person was immersed in my story, there was no getting off until the ride was over.

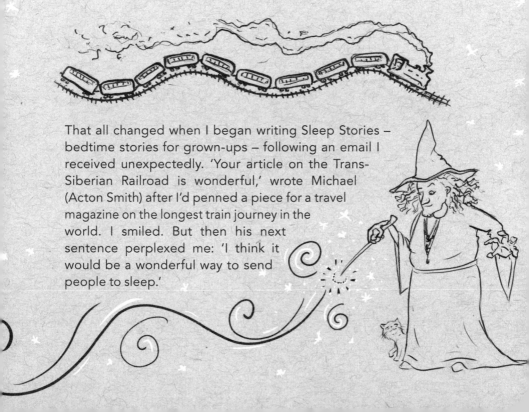

That all changed when I began writing Sleep Stories – bedtime stories for grown-ups – following an email I received unexpectedly. 'Your article on the Trans-Siberian Railroad is wonderful,' wrote Michael (Acton Smith) after I'd penned a piece for a travel magazine on the longest train journey in the world. I smiled. But then his next sentence perplexed me: 'I think it would be a wonderful way to send people to sleep.'

I wasn't sure if I should be insulted. For what kind of writer would I be if my words didn't grab and rouse but instead caused someone to nod off? The idea seemed crazy.

But sometimes an idea has a way of getting inside your thoughts and not letting go. Like a hex cast on me, the notion of Sleep Stories had me bewitched and, though I believed I wasn't going to take up the idea of writing one, I couldn't shake it off.

A few nights later I was looking after my friend's son. Just 2 years old, he was refusing to fall asleep – though he was clearly tired – and, feeling defeated, I offered to read him one of his books. He opted for a tale he loved – one about a friendly shark who lived on the Great Barrier Reef. What I noticed was that when I started he really wanted to stay awake until the end but, as I began reciting the words, I watched as his eyelids grew heavy and without even realizing it was happening he fell fast asleep.

It was then that it hit me – grown-ups can benefit from bedtime stories too. It's not dull writing. Rather, they allow us to escape into another world, one away from the bills, deadlines and concerns we have in our day-to-day lives.

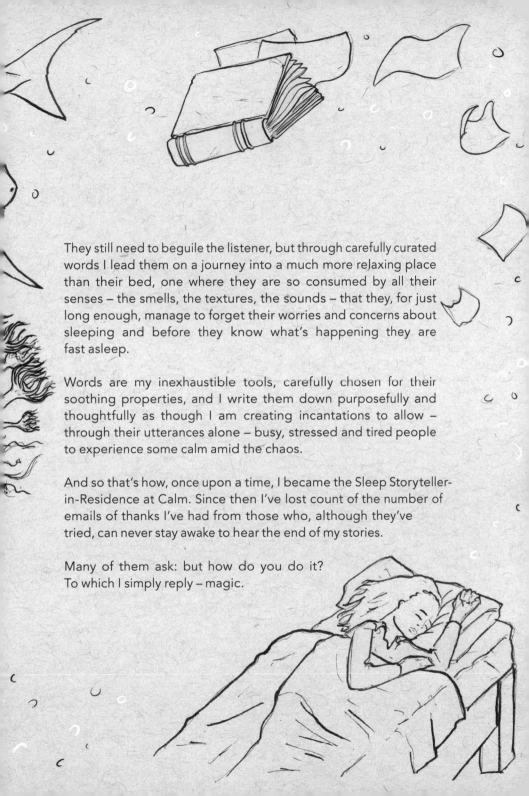

They still need to beguile the listener, but through carefully curated words I lead them on a journey into a much more relaxing place than their bed, one where they are so consumed by all their senses – the smells, the textures, the sounds – that they, for just long enough, manage to forget their worries and concerns about sleeping and before they know what's happening they are fast asleep.

Words are my inexhaustible tools, carefully chosen for their soothing properties, and I write them down purposefully and thoughtfully as though I am creating incantations to allow – through their utterances alone – busy, stressed and tired people to experience some calm amid the chaos.

And so that's how, once upon a time, I became the Sleep Storyteller-in-Residence at Calm. Since then I've lost count of the number of emails of thanks I've had from those who, although they've tried, can never stay awake to hear the end of my stories.

Many of them ask: but how do you do it?
To which I simply reply – magic.

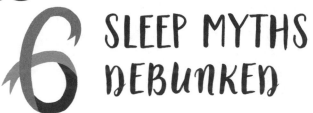

6 SLEEP MYTHS DEBUNKED

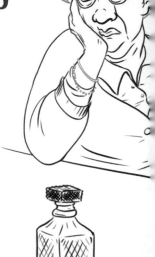

1 An alcoholic nightcap helps you sleep

A late-night slug of alcohol can help knock you out initially but studies show that alcohol actually impairs your deep sleep. Alcohol is also a diuretic, which means that drinking it makes you more likely to disrupt your sleep to visit the bathroom.

2 You can catch up on your sleep at the weekend

It might be tempting to sleep in at weekends after a sleep-deprived week but your body prefers a consistent sleeping pattern. 'Binge-sleeping' can upset your circadian rhythms and make things worse.

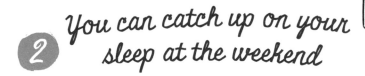

3 Snoring is harmless

If you are regularly snoring then you should see a doctor about it. Snoring could be a sign of poor airflow and sleep apnoea, which can result in reduced blood oxygen and heart problems. Frequent snoring can also be a sign of hypertension.

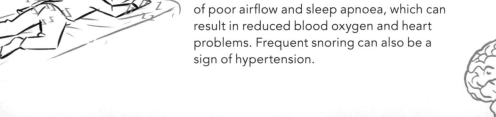

4 Older people need less sleep

It's true that sleep quality declines as we get older, with the result that we might take more naps as we age, but it's not true that we need less sleep when we're older. Older people need just as much sleep as before. Research also suggests that deep sleep can cut the risk of Alzheimer's disease.

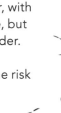

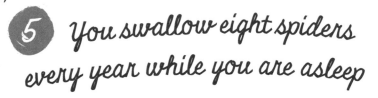

 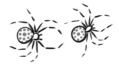

5 You swallow eight spiders every year while you are asleep

Arachnophobes can rest easy. It's very unlikely that you will swallow any spiders while you are asleep, as your body vibrates and makes enough noises while asleep to put off any eight-legged creatures wanting to crawl into your mouth.

6 It's dangerous to wake a sleepwalker

If you see a sleepwalker heading somewhere dangerous then stop them! Waking a sleepwalker will not give them a heart attack or kill them. It's best to walk a sleepwalker safely back to their bed – or else to make a noise from a safe distance away in order to wake them up.

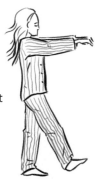

The Shipp

The most effective natural sleep aid ever?

Struggling to drift off? Let one of Britain's national institutions lull you to sleep with its soothing delivery of the Shipping Forecast. Yes, that's right. The Shipping Forecast.

First broadcast by the BBC in 1911, this prediction of weather that's vital for all seafarers around the coast of Britain is played four times a day – 00.48, 05.20, 12.01 and 17.54 – on BBC Radio 4 longwave. The iconic weather report is incomprehensible to most listeners with its strange and unfamiliar areas and numbers for wind speeds. But it turns out that this super-useful broadcast – never more than 380 words – is the perfect sedative to lull any late-night landlubbers into full-on slumber.

North   East   Viking   North   Utsire   Sou

Dogger   Fisher   German   Bight   Hum

Plymouth   Biscay   Trafalgar   FitzRoy   S

Rockall   Malin   Hebrides   Bailey

ing forecast

And now a new Sleep Story on Calm has capitalized on this uniquely British programme's soporific effect in 'And now the Shipping Forecast . . .' – a reinvented bedtime story for grown-ups, read by the familiar 'voice of the Shipping Forecast', former BBC announcer Peter Jefferson, who joined the BBC in 1964.

In the Sleep Story, Peter gives his own introduction and explains for the benefit of beginners the forecast's history, background and special place, if not cult status, in British life.

So, are you sitting comfortably? Then, we'll begin . . .

'And now the Shipping Forecast, issued by the Met Office on behalf of the Maritime and Coastguard Agency . . . The general synopsis . . .'

Utsire   Forties   Cromarty   Forth   Tyne

Thames   Dover   Wight   Portland

Lundy   Fastnet   Irish   Sea   Shannon

Isle   Faeroes   Southeast   Iceland

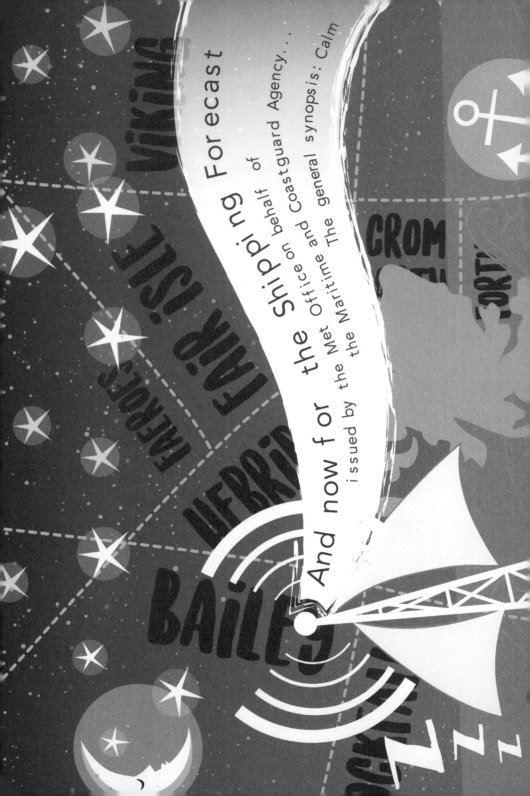

VIKING

FAIR ISLE

FAEROES

LIFBRID

BAILEY

CROM

FORT

And now for the Shipping Forecast issued by the Met Office on behalf of the Maritime and Coastguard Agency... The general synopsis: Calm

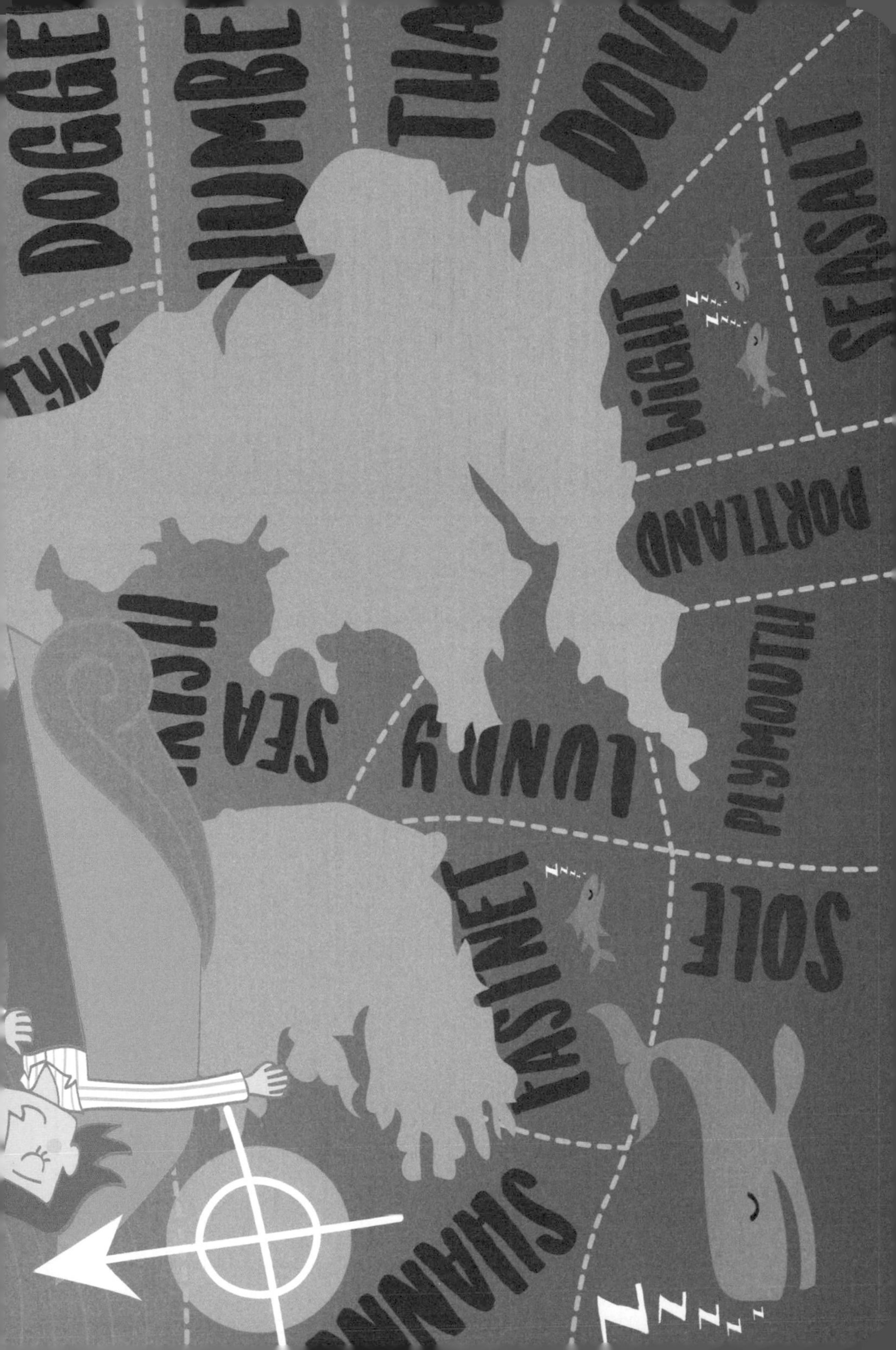
FASTNET
SOLE
LUNDY
SEA
PLYMOUTH
PORTLAND
WIGHT
SEASALT

DATE

WHAT MADE YOU FEEL CALM TODAY?

WHAT WERE THREE HIGHLIGHTS OF TODAY? ✦☽

Sleep intention diary

Let's start by checking in with you and your current sleep practices.

Here are some practices that can improve sleep quality. How many are part of your routine? Which are you not doing currently but feel doable and desirable to you?

Put a checkbox in the appropriate column for each:

Current practice | New habit to try |
--- | --- | ---
☐ | ☐ | Listening to a Sleep Story
☐ | ☐ | Doing deep sleep meditation
☐ | ☐ | Doing the evening wind down Calm body session
☐ | ☐ | Listening to relaxing music
☐ | ☐ | Dimming the lights
☐ | ☐ | Drinking lots of water during the day but not drinking too much right before bed
☐ | ☐ | Regular exercise
☐ | ☐ | Avoiding screens and blue light before bed

- ☐ ☐ Getting sunlight during the day
- ☐ ☐ Using a sleep mask
- ☐ ☐ Using earplugs
- ☐ ☐ Drinking decaffeinated tea before bed
- ☐ ☐ A scoop of coconut oil before bed
- ☐ ☐ A clutter-free bedroom
- ☐ ☐ Avoiding particular foods
- ☐ ☐ Keeping a notebook by your bed to empty your thoughts and to-do list on to paper so that you can rest your mind
- ☐ ☐ Meditation
- ☐ ☐ Breathing exercises
- ☐ ☐ Calm sleep mist
- ☐ ☐ Aromatherapy
- ☐ ☐ Cooler temperatures in the bedroom
- ☐ ☐ A set bedtime

A good laugh and a long sleep are the two BEST

Acknowledgements

This book is only in existence because of the hard work, ideas and inspiration of a very large group of extraordinary people. Alex Tew and I would like to say a huge and heartfelt thank you to every single one of them: I've been fortunate enough to work with Enes Alili for almost a decade and once again he's been able to weave his design magic through every part of this project. His boundless enthusiasm and long hours burning the midnight oil kept us all on track. Peter Freedman is a PR genius and has dreamed up endless sleep-related stories for Calm as well as contributed a huge amount to the book itself. Casey McKerchie has kept us all on track with his spreadsheets, enthusiasm and humour. Thanks to Nicholas Head, the Calm Exec Producer, for the dedication to his craft and for sparking over 100 Sleep Stories into life. Enes Alili for his cover ideas, boundless energy and world-class design skills. Alex Will for his friendship and brilliance in all areas of life (and Leo Will), Malcolm Scovil for his friendship and for organizing the very special book launch for our first book way back in 2015. To everyone on the Calm team who has made this rocket ship journey such a wild and fun ride: Dun Wang, Tyler Sheaffer, Katie Shill, Henderson Lafond and the rest of the team in SF and around the world.

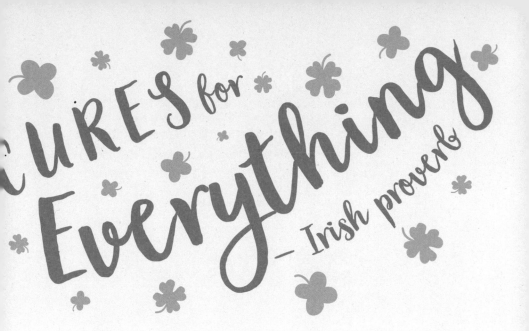

CURES for Everything
— Irish proverb

To all our investors who have believed in us. Susan MacTavish Best for her inspiration, salons and silver goblets, Sierra Acton Smith for her big smiles and sleepless nights, Clodagh Connell, Inna Semenyuk, Nicole Quinn, Shed Simove, Tom Boardman, Neil Porter, Vivienne Errington-Barnes, Matt Shone, Jamie Klingler, Michelle Dewberry, Charles Baybutt, Steve Cleverley, Oli Barrett, Colette Smith, Anna Acton, Ben Hull, Gracie Hull, Lana Hull. To my friends at Penguin, who have been calm, patient and brilliant: Venetia Butterfield, Marianne Tatepo, Emily Robertson, Nikki Sims, Natalie Wall, Josie Murdoch, Zoe Horn Haywood and Annie Lee. And in particular, my thanks to Tamara Levitt for creating and narrating such authentic, powerful and heartfelt meditations (and Sleep Stories) that have changed so many lives around the world. Alex and I would also like to thank all the fans of the Calm app and those of you who've bought the book. Welcome to the journey and please get involved. We'd love to hear your thoughts and feedback, so you're very welcome to join the community online (@calm) or connect with Alex (@tewy) and myself (@acton) on Twitter.

sleep glossary

adenosine a chemical compound that starts building in your bloodstream from the moment you wake up until bedtime.

CBT-I behavioural therapy targeting insomnia issues in particular.

circadian rhythm a roughly 24-hour inbuilt clock.

endorphins 'feel good' neurotransmitters.

ghrelin hormone that stimulates hunger.

leptin chemical that conveys fullness.

melatonin hormone that signals to your body and brain that it's dark and time to sleep.

NREM sleep non rapid eye movement sleep, or 'dreamless' sleep (stages 1, 2, 3).

oxytocin the 'love hormone'.

polyphasic sleep sleep on several occasions within 24 hours.

prolactin hormone that makes you feel relaxed and sleepy.

proprioceptive system our body's sensory receptor.

REM sleep rapid eye movement, the phase of sleep with more bodily movement and faster pulse and breathing (the phase that precedes stages 1 to 3 of the sleep cycle).

sleep drive a measure of a person's biological need for sleep.

sleep latency the time it takes you to nod off.

suprachiasmatic nucleus an area of your brain that sits behind your eyes – and serves as your 24-hour rhythm generator.

vasopressin hormone that stops you needing the loo at night and is associated with sleep.

Grateful acknowledgement is made by the publisher for permission to reproduce the images on the following pages:

Alamy: 146, 148, 214; © Ana Yael: 101; Deina Abigail Diaz: 162–3; Enes Alili: 26, 56–9, 92–3, 142–3, 170–71, 220–21, 226; © Federica Bordoni: 74–5, 178–9; Getty Images: 18–23, 90, 116, 119, 124, 144, 149–150, 154, 182–3, 215, 240; © Katie Rose Johnston: 176–7, 202–3; © Harriet Lee-Merrion: 166–7; 180–81; Freepik.com: 40, 52–3, 69, 78–9, 83, 88–9, 100, 104, 125–9, 135, 173, 214, 216–17, 229; James Balance: 46–9, 54–5 (background), 85, 90, 222–7; iStock: 64, 106; imageafter: 206–7; Neil Tony Porter (illustrator): 6, 111, 130; Pexels: 14, 105; © Penelope Dullaghan: 86–7; Shutterstock: 7, 32–5, 50–51, 66, 96, 102, 114, 120–121, 138–9, 156, 188–9, 212, 218; Sierra Acton Smith (picture): 76; Unsplash: 8–11, 28, 30, 44, 45, 60–63, 81, 82, 84, 98–9, 108–9, 113, 122–3, 136–7, 145, 158–9, 160, 165, 169, 184, 185, 187, 192–4, 204–5, 214, 234–5, 238–9; Wikipedia, © James Cameron: 46; Wikipedia: 7, 24–5, 45, 110, 161; Zoe Horn Haywood: 31, 52–3, 68, 70–71, 94–6, 132–4, 164, 172, 174–5, 195–9, 219, 228–9.

Sources:

Center for Environmental Therapeutics: 46–9; *New Scientist*: 72; National Sleep Foundation: 77, 97, 140–41; *Sunday Times*: 113.

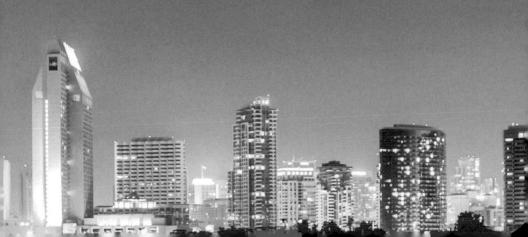

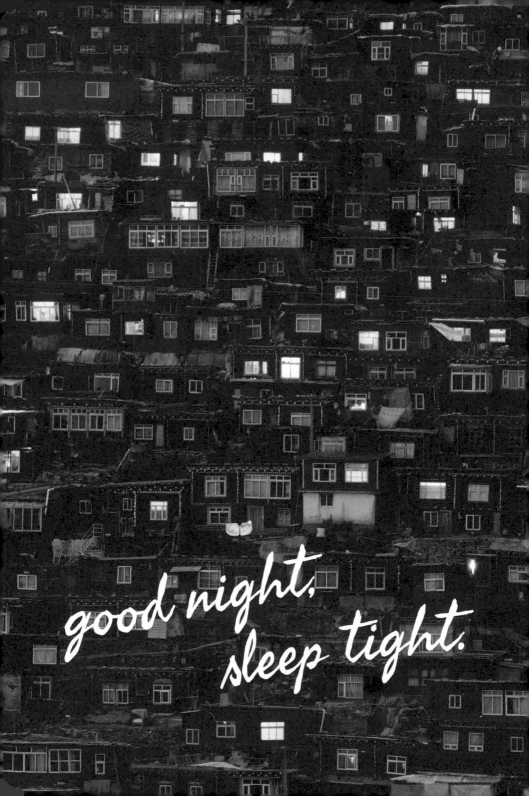